LESSER KNOWN GERMPLASM OF SMALL RUMINANTS

LESSER KNOWN GERMPLASM OF SMALL RUMINANTS

N. Ramachandran
S. P. Singh
S. K. Jindal
A.K. Goel
P. K. Rout

ICAR-Central Institute for Research on Goats
Makhdoom, Farah-281 122 (Mathura), India

SSPH

SATISH SERIAL PUBLISHING HOUSE
403, Express Tower, Commercial Complex
Azadpur, Delhi-110033 (India)
Phone : 011-27672852, Fax : 91-11-27672046
e-mail : info@satishserial.com, hkjain1975@yahoo.com
Website : www.satishserial.com

Published by :

SATISH SERIAL PUBLISHING HOUSE

403, Express Tower, Commercial Complex, Azadpur, Delhi-110033 (INDIA)
Phone : 011-27672852 Fax : 91-11-27672046
E-mail : info@satishserial.com, hkjain1975@yahoo.com

ISBN 978-93-85055-78-2

Composed, Designed & Printed in India

Preface

Goats and sheep are being seen as the 'Future Animal' for sustaining livelihood and nutritional security of the small and marginal farmers and landless labourers, apart from production of meat and milk on commercial lines to substantially meet the ever increasing demands of milk and meat in India. The importance of goat milk lies in its nutritive and medicinal properties and of the goat meat in its leaner composition with no religious taboos against its consumption. Goats and sheep are widely adapted and can thrive well and reproduce in all climatic conditions of the country and are being reared under Extensive, Semi-Intensive and Intensive systems of management. The production performance varies widely depending upon the inputs available under different systems of rearing. The Extensive system of goat rearing is being switched over to Semi-Intensive and Intensive management systems as an outcome of shrinking grazing land and increased preference towards commercial goat farming.

India possesses 24 defined goat and 40 sheep breeds spread across the country accounting for only nearly one-third of the total population. The majority of the small ruminant population in India are lesser known, non-descript or unrecognized but they are well known for their production potential and adaptability. It has been observed that sheep and goat farming as a livelihood enterprise is shifting to commercial enterprise and the transportation stress as well as poor foundation stock are the hurdles in running a viable enterprise for longer period. At this juncture, the knowledge on the performance of few lesser known goat and sheep germplasm will help the rearers to focus and buy the breeds available in nearby locations to avoid such initial losses.

The authors have compiled the sizable information on a large number of lesser known goat germplasm published already in the literature for the use of all concerned in goat rearing. The use of information, data and pictures throughout the document with proper references aptly acknowledged. The authors are sure that the information contained in this book will be very useful to entrepreneur, research scholars, teachers, scientists engaged with small ruminant improvement programmes and commercial sheep and goat farming.

Authors

ABOUT THE AUTHORS

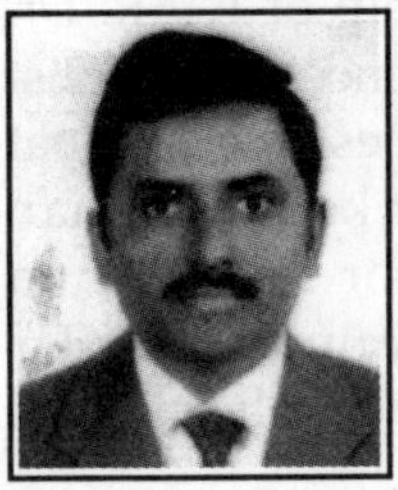

Dr. N. Ramachandran, Ph.D. is currently working as Senior Scientist (Livestock Production and Management) at ICAR-Central Institute for Research on Goats, Makhdoom, Mathura. He obtained his M.V. Sc. degree from National Dairy Research Institute, Karnal, Haryana and Ph.D. degree in Animal Science from Dr. Bhimrao Ambedkar University (Formerly Agra University), Agra in the year of 2000 and 2012, respectively. He joined Agriculture Research Service (ARS) of ICAR as a Scientist in 2003, obtained 4 months FOCARS training at National Academy of Agricultural Research and Management (NAARM), Hyderabad, thereafter joined ICAR-Central Institute for Research on Goats, Makhdoom, Mathura. Dr. Ramachandran obtained specialized foreign training on "New Techniques for Sustainable Sheep and Goat Production" at Amman, Jordan in 2014, jointly sponsored by International Centre for Agricultural Research in Dry Areas (ICARDA) and Japan International Cooperation Agency (JICA). He has more than thirteen years research experience in the field of Goat Production and Management with specialization in the area of Livestock Shelters, Andrology and Managemental interventions to improve productivity of animals. Dr Ramachandran is the Editor of "CIRG News" from 2011. He has 5 International and 20 National research publications, 35 chapters in different books/compendiums, 2 books/manuals in his credit.

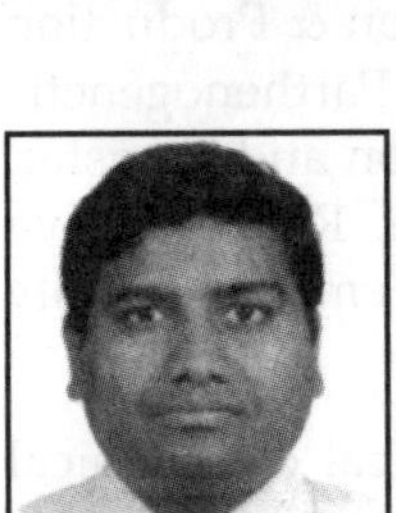

Dr. S.P. Singh, Ph.D. (University of Bonn, Germany), is a Scientist of Animal Physiology, presently working in the Division of Physiology, Reproduction and Shelter Management at Central Institute for Research on Goats, Makhdoom, Farah, Mathura (U.P.). He graduated in Veterinary Science and Animal Husbandry in 2004 from Veterinary College, NDUAT, Faizabad and completed his M.V.Sc. in 2006 from IVRI, Izatnagar. He has presently 16 research papers to his credit including 9 in International Journals of high impact factor. He has a good international exposure to participate trainings, seminars, conferences etc. in USA, Denmark, Norway, Switzerland, Italy and Germany.

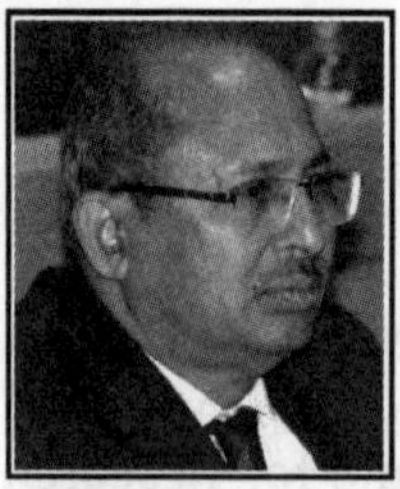

Dr. S.K. Jindal, Ph.D. Acting Director at ICAR-Central Institute for Research on Goats, Makhdoom, Mathura. Dr. Jindal obtained his Masters and Ph.D. degree from National Dairy Research Institute, Karnal. He was recipient of Senior Research Fellowship of ICAR. Dr. Jindal has more than 38 years of experience as a scientist in the field of livestock production especially goat production. Dr. Jindal earlier worked at Indian Veterinary Research Institute and Central Institute for Research on Buffaloes. Dr. Jindal visited several Universities in USA under Indo-US programme. He has published 5 books and more than 100 publications in National and International Journals of repute.

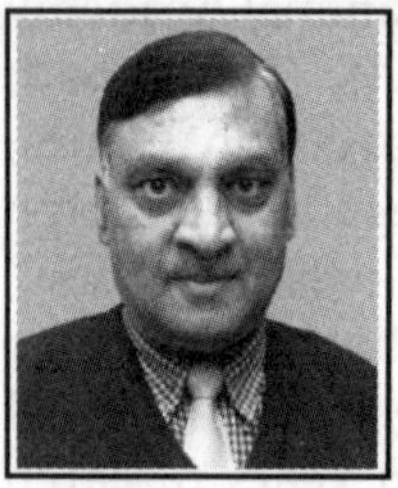

Dr. A.K. Goel, Ph.D. is a research scientist in the area of Reproductive Biotechnology in Small Ruminants. Dr. Goel is presently serving as Principal Scientist (Animal Reproduction) in ICAR - Central Institute for Research on Goats, Makhdoom, Mathura (UP). Dr. Goel graduated in Veterinary Science and Animal Husbandry and completed Master's degree in Veterinary Obstetrics & Gynaecology from College of Veterinary Science & Animal Husbandry, Mathura in the year of 1980 and 1982, respectively. He completed his Ph.D. degree from Dr. B. R. Ambedkar University (Formerly Agra University) Agra in 1998 for his work on ETT in goats.

He has been associated in diversified areas of Research, Teaching, Training and Extension Activities in Small Ruminant Reproduction & Production for more than 3 decades. His area of work includes, ETT, Parthenogenetic Embryo Production, *In-vitro* & *In-vivo* Embryo Production and Transfer, Application of Imaging Techniques in Reproduction, Reproductive Physiology/ Endocrinology, Semen Cryo-preservation, Female Infertility & Transfer of Viable Technologies.

He has published 105 Research Papers, Reviews, Clinical & Technical Articles in Peer Reviewed Journals of National and International repute and presented 144 Research Papers including 20 lead papers in various National & International Scientific gatherings. He has also published 11 Technical Bulletins and 43 Popular Articles. He has Authored /Edited 08 Books and Laboratory Manual. Dr. Goel has contributed 46 Book Chapters in many referred Publications on Goat Production and Reproduction and Climate Change. He has provisionally patented one Technology. He has guided 1 doctorate and 6 master's degrees students. He visited USA to acquire advance trainings in embryo technology and ultrasonography. He is also associated as life member of 16 professional/scientific societies, besides serving as Vice President of ISSGPU and Associate Editor of Indian Journal of Small Ruminants. He is recipient of ISSGPU Fellow Award-2012 (FISSGPU) of The Indian Society for Sheep and Goat Production and Utilization, ISSAR Fellow Award- 2013 (FISSAR) of The Indian Society for the Study of Animal Reproduction and Special Recognition Award 2008-09 of Mobilization- Society for Community Mobilization for Sustainable Development, New Delhi.

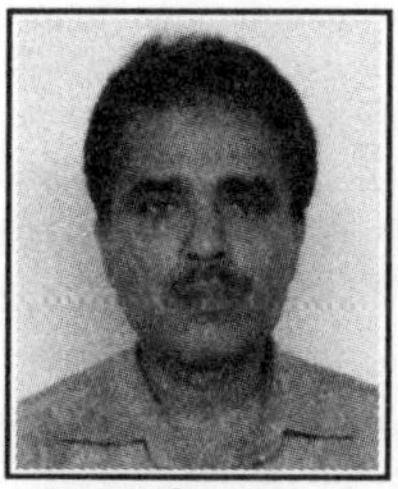

Dr. Pramod K. Rout, Ph.D. is presently working as Principal Scientist and Project coordinator, AICRP on goat improvement at ICAR - Central Institute for Research on Goats, Makhdoom, Mathura under Indian Council of Agricultural Research, New Delhi. He is a graduate in Veterinary Science from college of Veterinary Sciences and Animal Husbandry, Bhubaneswar and completed his Master's and Doctoral degrees from Indian Veterinary Research Institute, Izatnagar, Bareilly. He has worked as post-doctoral fellow at Roslin Institute, University of Edinburgh, Scotland, UK. His field of specialization is Genetics of Disease Resistance and improvement and conservation of Goat genetic resources.

Dr. Rout has made outstanding contribution to the areas of Genetics of disease resistance, Genetic diversity of livestock and Conservation of animal genetic resources. He was responsible to establish genetic origin of Indian goats and suggested new insight into the origin of Indian goat breeds and their probable domestication. His work on milk proteome analysis established that Indian goats are carrying better allelic combination for protein yield with respect to European goats. He has also worked in the area of conservation of endangered goats in their natural habitat with active participation of farmers under All India Coordinated Research Project. He has made significant contribution by initiating molecular studies in goat biology. He has been involved in wide range of professional activities such as teaching, guiding doctoral, M.V.Sc. and M.Sc. students and extension works. He has been invited by different national and international organizations to contribute lead papers in different seminars and symposia. He has guided 4 Ph.D. and 14 M.V.Sc. and M.Sc. students. He has published more than 75 research paper and 28 chapters in different books/compendiums.

Contents

Chapter 1

INTRODUCTION

Small ruminants play an important role in the development of rural economy of India. Small ruminant rearing significantly contributes to the livelihood security of poor farmers, even under challenging environmental conditions as inadequate rainfall, very high temperatures and poor soil fertility, wherein crop cultivation is often difficult. Small ruminants not only contribute to the household livelihood and nutrition security, but are also a hedge against the losses in agriculture consequent upon adverse climatic conditions. The total number of households and household enterprises, both rural and urban, which rear sheep and goats are 4.55 and 33.01 million respectively. Together, the goat and sheep rearing households constitute 15% of the total number of households in the country (19th Livestock Census, 2012).

Goat is one of the important farm animals which have been domesticated by man since time immemorial and has been a traditional occupation of marginal farmers and landless labourers. Goat is known as the 'poor man's cow' in India and as 'wet nurse' of infants in Europe. Goat significantly contributes to the agrarian economy and plays a vital role in the livelihood security of the small and marginal farmers in the country. Goats can be profitably raised with low investment under intensive as well as most extensive forms of grazing. Goat rearing is the best choice for the rural people in the country because of their wider adaptability, low investment, high fertility and fecundity, low feed and management needs, high feed conversion efficiency, quick pay off and low risk involved. Goats can be kept with little expense. Marginal or undulating lands, unsuitable for other types of livestock, may be used and any inexpensive shelter will suffice. Goats have good production potential even under hostile physical environment and sparse browsing resources. It is a known fact that of all the domestic animals, goat doubtless has greatest range of adaptation (Jindal, 1984). Sheep are reared in relatively larger herds (average 60-70 animals per herd) whereas goats are reared in smaller numbers, ranging from 1-10, on average. Goat rearing is also characterized by a greater involvement of women, and hence offers an opportunity for empowerment of women through goat-based livelihood improvement. India supports 16.1% of the world's goat population and 6.4% of sheep population (FAO Statistics, 2013), making it among the highest livestock holding countries in the world. Out of total livestock population of the country (512.05 million), 26.4 % is contributed by the goats (135.17 million) and 12.7% is contributed by sheep (65.06 million), (19th Livestock Census, 2012). The annual population growth rate of goats in India has varied from about 0.94% to about 5.13% with an average of 3.55% during 1951-2009, although, about 47.5 million goats making about 40% of the total population are slaughtered for meat every year. However, the Goat population has declined recently by 3.82% over the previous census (140.54 million in 2007 vs 135.17 million in 2012). Similarly, the sheep population has also shown a declining trend (9.07%) during the same period.

India produced 43.90% of the milk, 16.03% of the meat and 18.78% of the fresh skins of the production in Asia and 25.76% of the milk, 11.35% of the meat and 14.13% of the fresh skins of the world production. The analysis shows that goats contribute nearly 4% and 16 % of total milk (5.048 million tonns) and meat (0.970 million tonns) production of the country, respectively, whereas, the sheep contributes about 7% (0.441 million tonns) of total meat production of country (Basic Animal Husbandry and Fisheries Statistics, 2014). The state with the highest number of goats is Rajasthan (21.6 million), followed by Uttar Pradesh (15.6 million). Eastwhile Andhra Pradesh has highest number of sheep population (26.935 million), followed by Karnataka (9.583 million). The meat production from goat is highest in the State of West Bengal with 0.242 million tonnes per year. The second and third highest average production of meat are reported by Uttar Pradesh (0.184 million tonnes) and Andhra Pradesh (0.087 million tonnes), respectively (Basic Animal Husbandry and Fisheries Statistics, 2014). The goat sector in India generates about 4.2% rural employment and around 22.5 million families belonging to small and marginal farmers and landless labourers are engaged in goat farming (FAO, 2010).

Over centuries, livestock population/animal kingdom has been divided into a number of subpopulations i.e. **species** and breeds within a species, because of geographical isolation, selection by their human keepers and other evolutionary forces. Each species is further subdivided in to sub species or breeds. In general, **breed** can be defined as 'a group of animals of the same species having same origin (related by descent) and having common characteristics like general appearance, body color and size, configuration etc. Breed as adopted by FAO is defined as either a sub specific group of domestic livestock with definable and identifiable external characteristics that enable it to be separated by visual appraisal from other similarly defined groups within the same species or a group for which geographical and/or cultural separation from phenotypically similar groups has led to acceptance of its separate identity (FAO, 1999). The breed is further subdivided in to **strains** based on isolation from each other due to geographical conditions or due to different aims of breeding the animals. The **strain** is further subdivided in to **lines** in which the individuals of a breed/strain are more closely related to each other's due to interbreeding.

The goat was domesticated first among all ruminants during Neolithic age along with the cultivation of cereals sometime before 7000 B.C. at the slopes of the Zagros Mountains on the borders of presently Iran and Iraq. According to Mason (1988), the ancestor of the present breeds of goat is *Capra hircus* and *C. aegagrus* - the Bezoar goat. This sub species is distributed from Sind in the East through Iran and Asia Minor to Crete and the Cyclades in the West. The origin and development of goat breeds in Indian sub-continent is not clearly known, although the remains of goat along with other animals like dog, buffalo, sheep and pig have been reported from the Neotitive site excavation in the districts of Hoshnagsabed. The Harappa toys demonstrate the representation of a goat and two seals from Mohenjo-daro show the wild bezoar goat with enormous curled horns, and a bearded domestic male goat with side-spreading horns. The goats of hircus species reached undivided Indian subcontinent from the Western Asia by North-Western and North-Eastern routes between 7500-7000 B.C. But it is strongly believed that the present breeds have evolved from the cross of hircus species brought to India along with Muslim invasions up to the 14th Century. Crossbreeding with European breeds has been sporadically admitted in different pockets of India and claims have been made for development of a breed or strain.

In India, there are 24 goat breeds and 40 sheep breeds are recognized and the accession numbers have been assigned by the National Bureau of Animal Genetic Resources, Karnal (www.nbagr.res.in/reggoat.html). However, the variation in number of breeds is reported by various other agencies like FAO, DAHD etc. Besides these descript breeds, a major proportion of small ruminant population is constituted by the so called "non-descript" animals which do not conform to any of the described breeds. However, among these animals, there may be some groups of true breeding animals which remained ignored due to lack of systematic efforts for their description, documentation and improvement. According to the 2007 census about 63% of the total goat population are 'non-descript' or 'unrecognized'.

Diversity in sheep and goats is related with the geography and ecology of the region, environmental variations, production system and genetic potential of the breed. Several economically useful breeds have been developed with special adaptation features over the years to survive and simultaneously give sustained production under the various agro-climatic conditions of their habitat. Goats of temperate Himalayan region (Changthangi and Chegu) possess the finest quality under-coat called cashmere or pashmina. The goat breeds found in north and north-western region viz. Jamunapari, Marwari, Zalawadi, Beetal, Kutchi, Sirohi, Barbari, Mehsana, Surti, Jahkrana and Gohilwadi are primarily used for meat and milk purpose. In the southern and peninsular part of India, goats with dual production of meat and milk viz. Sangamneri, Osmanabadi, Kanni Adu, Malabari and Attapady Black are found. The highly prolific meat breed like Black Bengal goats are found in the Eastern region. Similarly, sheep breeds in different agro-ecological region of India also adapted to local weather conditions and produce mutton, wool, skin, manure etc.

There is a fair scope to identify, characterize and evaluate the existing small ruminant germplasm found in different parts of the country. Efforts are being made by researchers to document lesser known goat and sheep germplasm, which are not recognized till date. Although main stream breeds stem from local breeds, the major factor driving the livestock sector are often a threat for less competitive and marginalized local breeds. Verma *et al.* (2010) stated that in the era of intellectual property rights, proper documentation on such unexplored populations is essentially required. For this, these lesser known goat and sheep populations need to be studied intensively for their morphological traits and performance potential. The complete characterization (phenotypic and genetic) of these populations may indicate their distinctness of some or all of these populations. The genetic characterization using microsatellites or any other tool will reveal their genetic relationship with the descript animals of their native or neighbouring region. After confirming such distinctness, the population can be granted the breed status and the useful characteristics of the breed can be utilized for upgrading other non-descript populations. The information can also be utilized for formulating the breeding and conservation policy to improve the production of poor performing sheep and goats.

Though the sporadic reports are available from different state governments/NGOs on few less known sheep and goat germplasm, the compiled information on this aspect is not available for ready reference. Hence an attempt has been made after compiling the available information (farm, field) in literature to provide comprehensive information on the less known goat germplasm of India. The list of lesser known germplasm of sheep is also being included for the knowledge of small ruminant keepers in this book.

MAP overleaf

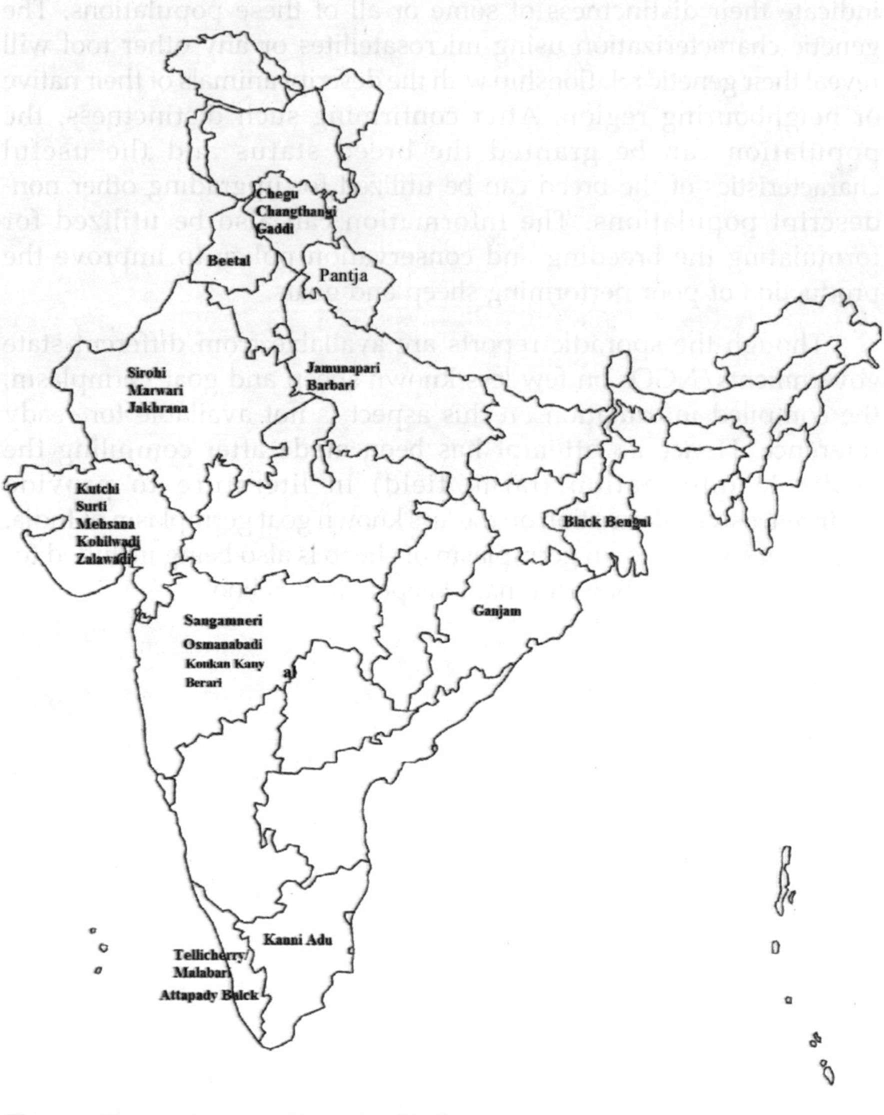

Figure : Recognized goat breeds of India

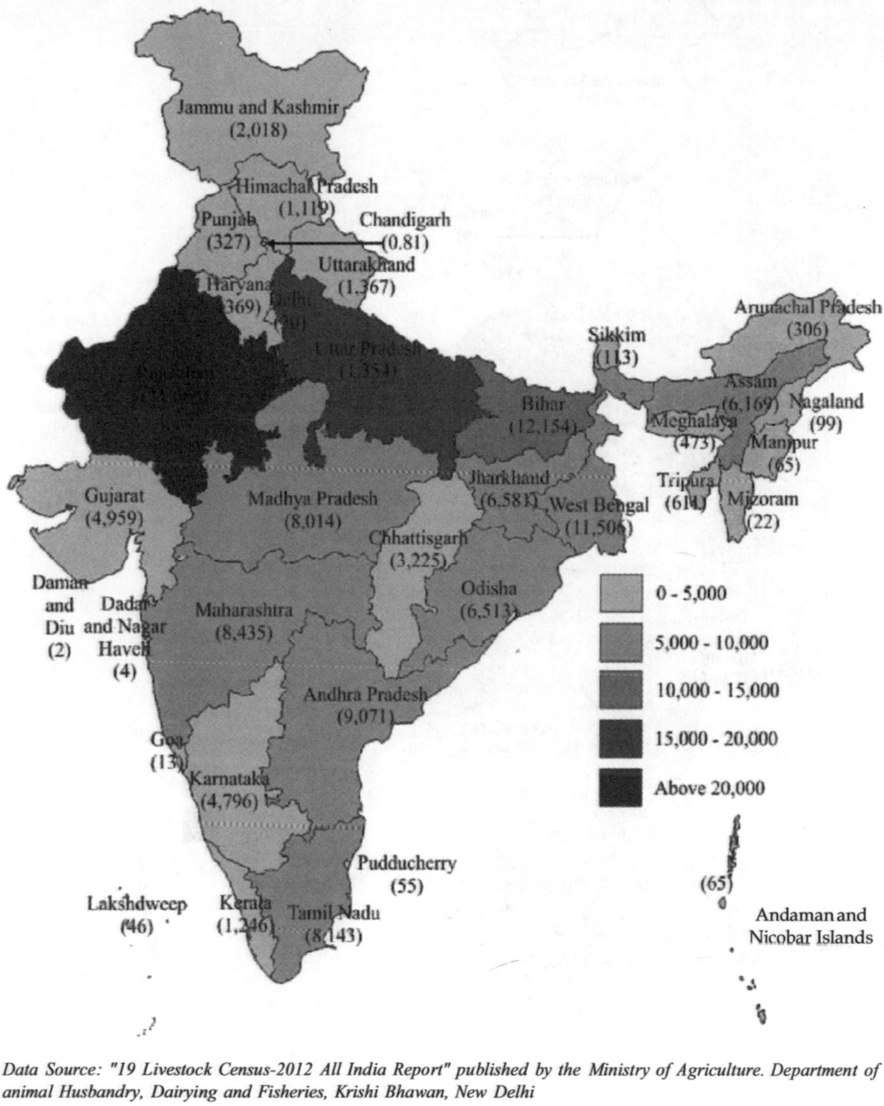

Data Source: "19 Livestock Census-2012 All India Report" published by the Ministry of Agriculture. Department of animal Husbandry, Dairying and Fisheries, Krishi Bhawan, New Delhi

Figure : Goat Population in India [19th Livestock Census, 2012 (all figures in 000)] South Asia Pro-Poor Livestock policy Programme, a joint initiative of NDDB and FAO (http://sapplpp.org/)

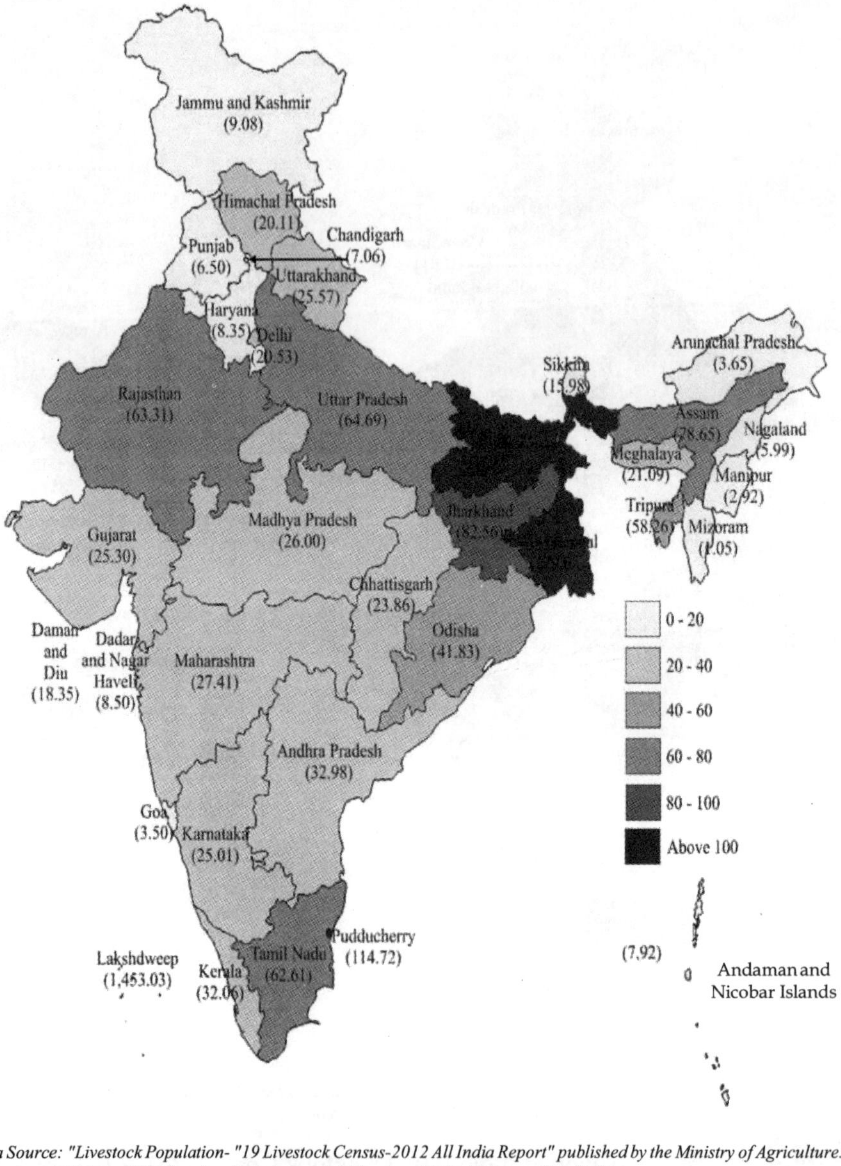

Data Source: "Livestock Population- "19 Livestock Census-2012 All India Report" published by the Ministry of Agriculture. Department of Animal Husbandry, Dairying and Fisheries, Krishi Bhawan, New Delhi
Area in sq km-http://en.wikipedia.org/wiki/List_of_states_and_union_territories_of_India_by_population

Figure : Population Density of Goats in India [19th Livestock Census, 2012 (numbers per sq km)] South Asia Pro-Poor Livestock policy Programme, a joint initiative of NDDB and FAO (http://sapplpp.org/)

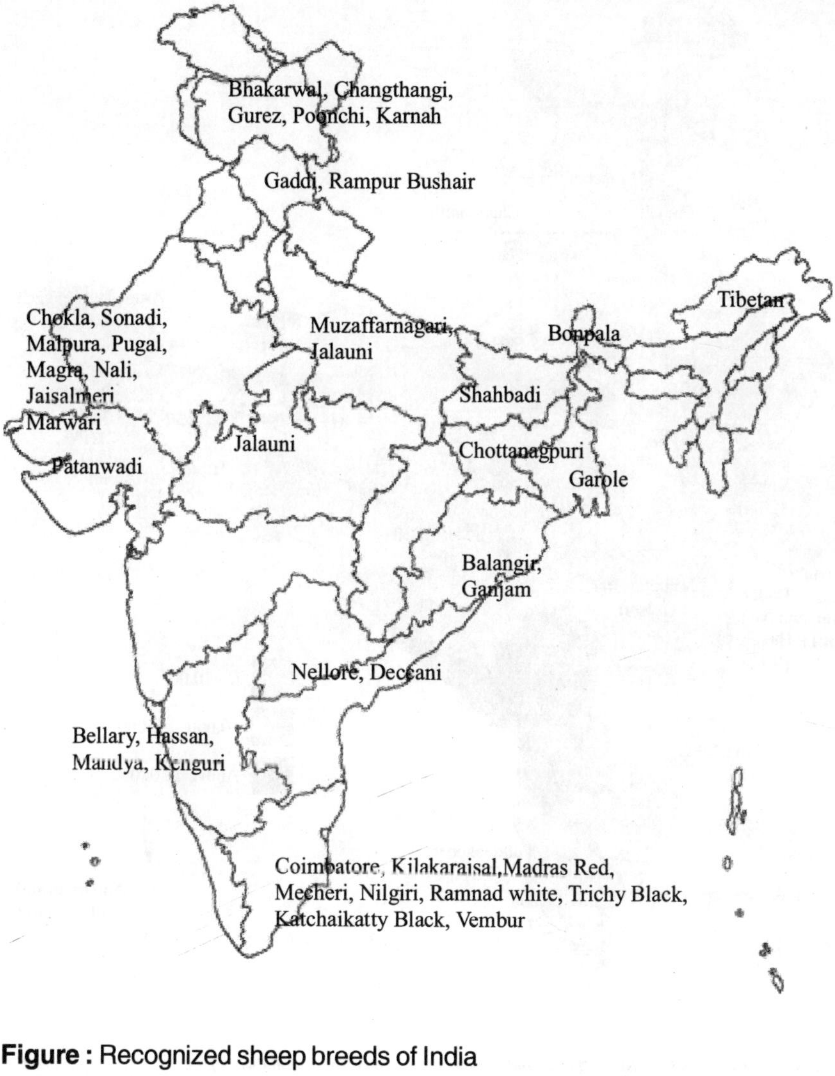

Figure : Recognized sheep breeds of India

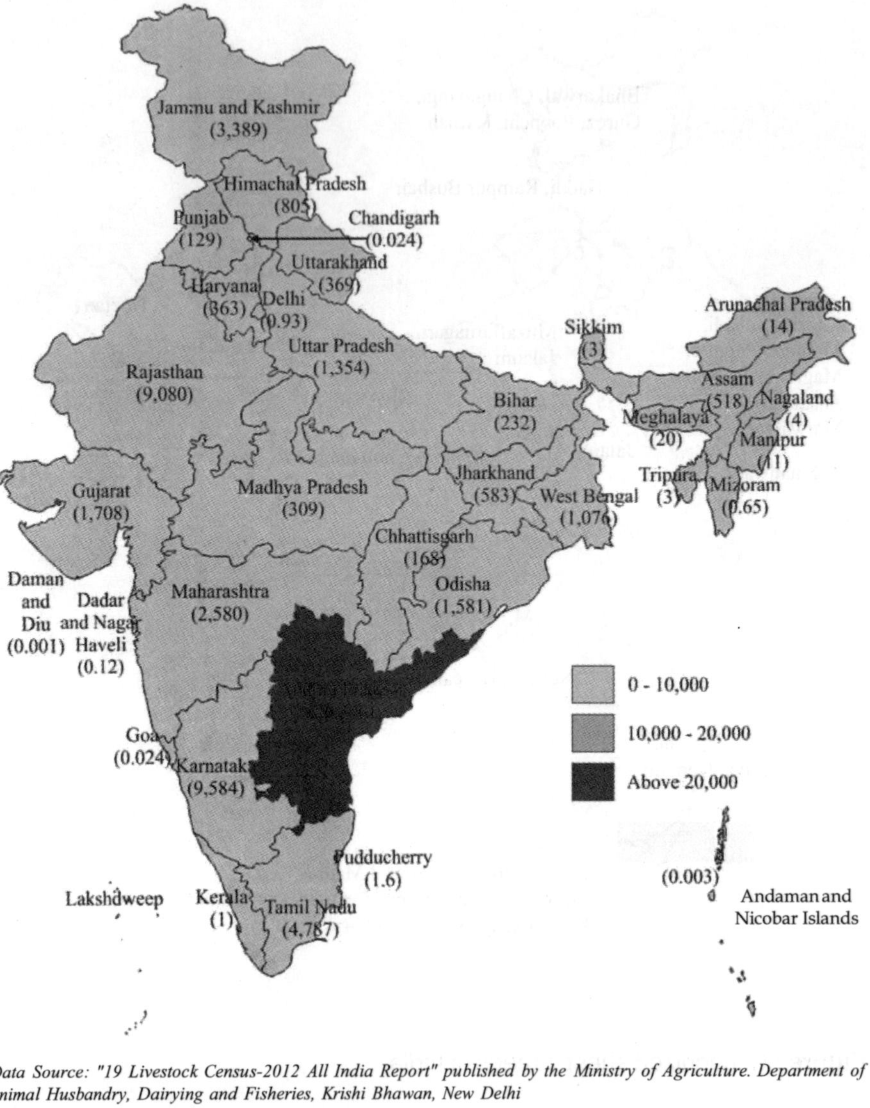

Data Source: "19 Livestock Census-2012 All India Report" published by the Ministry of Agriculture. Department of animal Husbandry, Dairying and Fisheries, Krishi Bhawan, New Delhi

Figure : Sheep Population in India [19th Livestock Census, 2012 (all figures in 000)] http://sapplpp.org/sheep-goat-poultry-statistics / common-resources / sheep-population-in-india#.VsqYxfl97IU

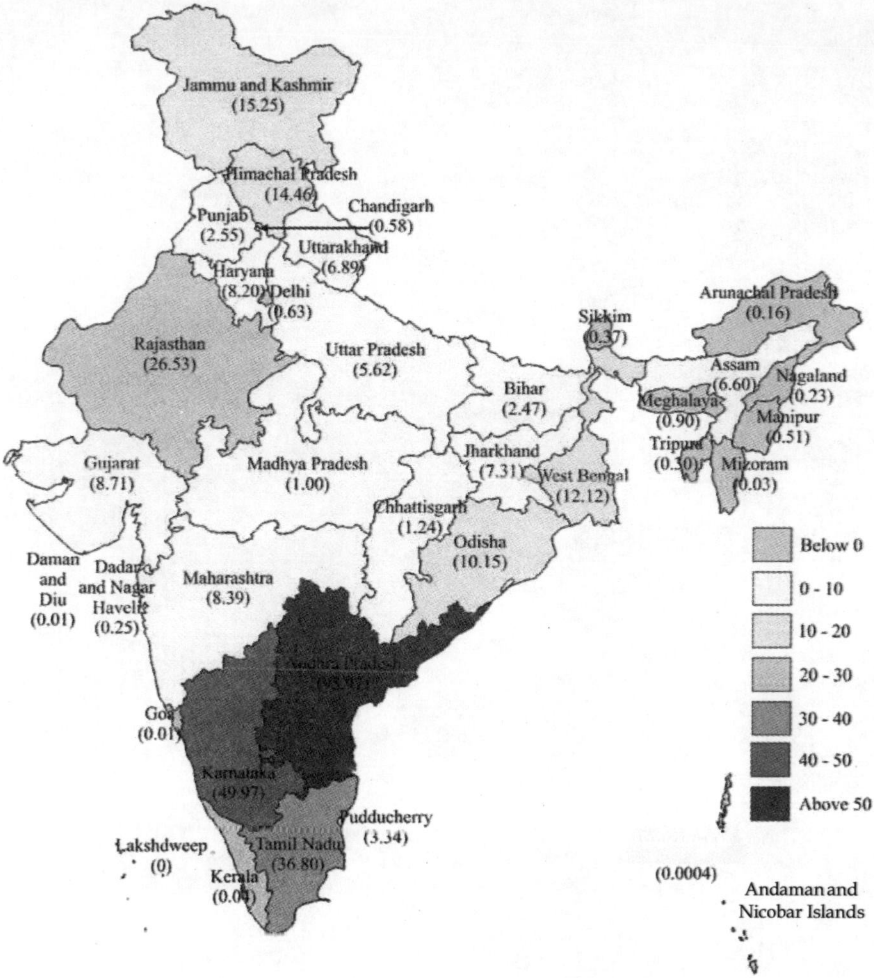

Data Source: "Livestock Population- "19 Livestock Census-2012 All India Report" published by the Ministry of Agriculture. Department of Animal Husbandry, Dairying and Fisheries, Krishi Bhawan, New Delhi
Area in sq km-http://en.wikipedia.org/wiki/List_of_states_and_union_territories_of_India_by_population

Figure : Population Density of Sheep in India [19th Livestock Census, 2012 (numbers persq km)] http://sapplpp.org/sheep-goat-poultry-statistics/common-resources/population-density-of-sheep-in-india#.VsqbEPl97IU

Chapter 2

LIST OF RECOGNIZED GOAT BREEDS IN INDIA

S. No.	Name	Home Tract	Body size	Utility	Image
1.	Attapady	Kerala	Medium	Meat	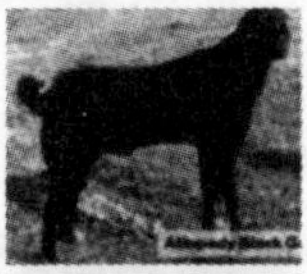
2.	Barbari	Uttar Pradesh and Rajasthan	Medium	Milk and meat	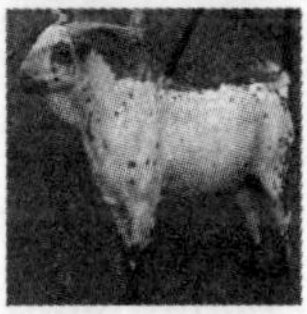
3.	Beetal	Punjab	Large	Milk and meat	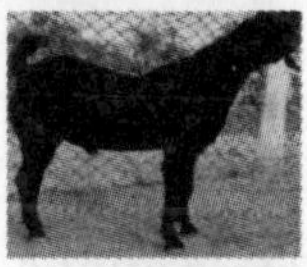
4.	Berari	Maharashtra	Medium	Meat	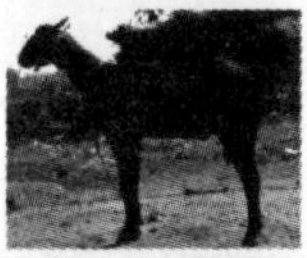
5.	Black Bengal	West Bengal	Small	Meat	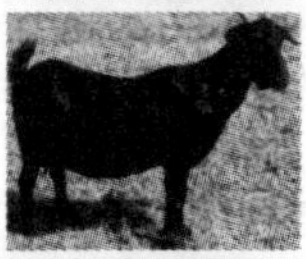
6.	Changthangi	Jammu and Kashmir	Small	Meat and fiber	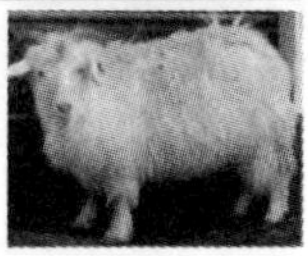

7.	Chegu	Himachal Pradesh	Small	Meat and fiber	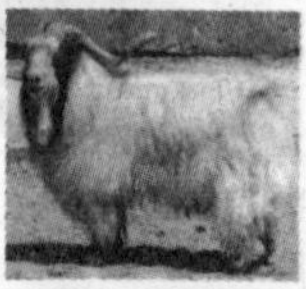
8.	Gaddi	Himachal Pradesh	Medium	Meat and fiber	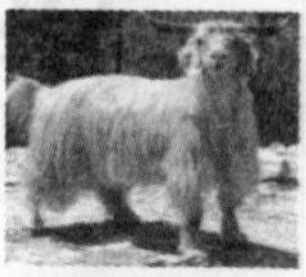
9.	Ganjam	Odisha	Medium	Meat	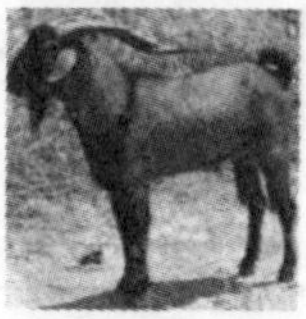
10.	Gohilwadi	Gujarat	Large	Meat and milk	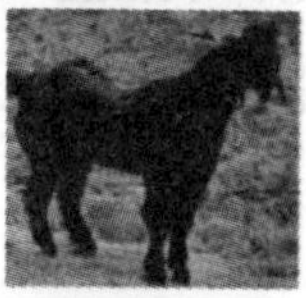
11.	Jakhrana	Rajasthan	Large	Milk and meat	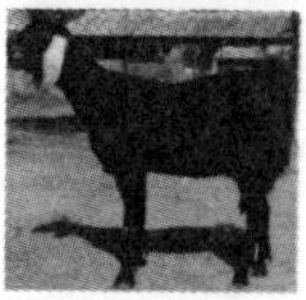
12.	Jamunapari	Uttar Pradesh	Large	Milk and meat	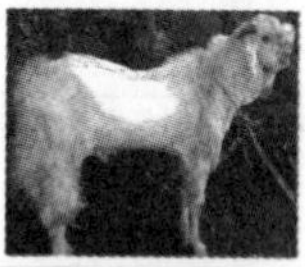
13.	Kanni Adu	Tamil Nadu	Medium	Meat	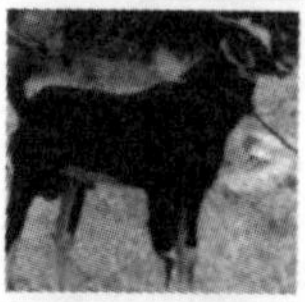
14.	Konkan Kanyal	Maharashtra	Medium	Meat	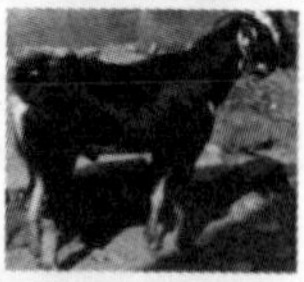
15.	Kutchi	Gujarat	Medium	Meat and milk	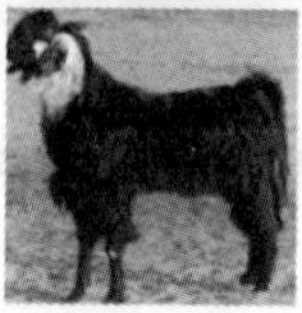

16.	Malabari	Kerala	Medium	Meat	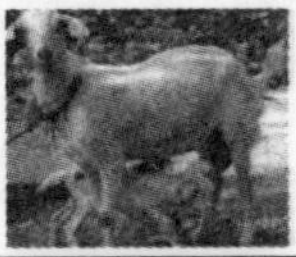
17.	Marwari	Rajasthan	Medium	Meat and fiber	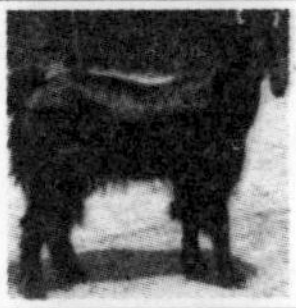
18.	Mehsana	Gujarat	Medium	Meat and milk	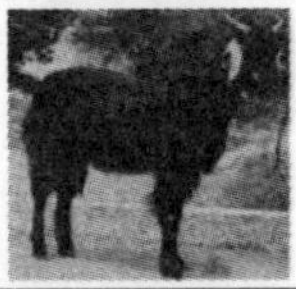
19.	Osmanabadi	Maharashtra	Medium	Meat and milk	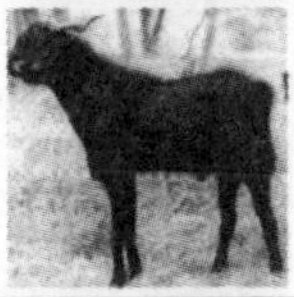
20.	Pantja	Uttarakhand and Uttar Pradesh	Medium	Meat and milk	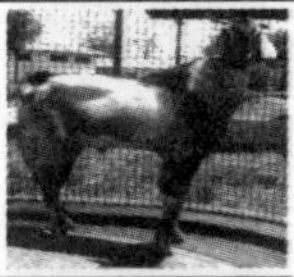
21.	Sangamneri	Maharashtra	Medium	Meat and milk	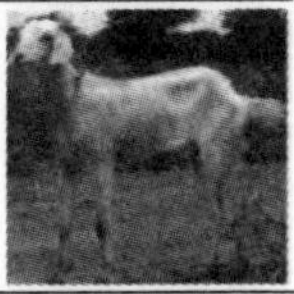
22.	Sirohi	Rajasthan and Gujarat	Large	Milk and meat	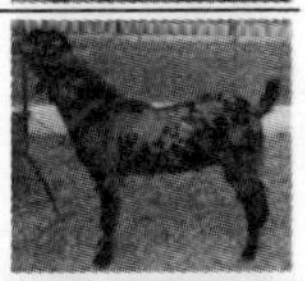
23.	Surti	Gujarat	Medium	Milk and meat	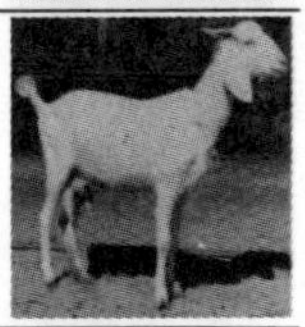
24.	Zalawadi	Gujarat	Medium	Meat and milk	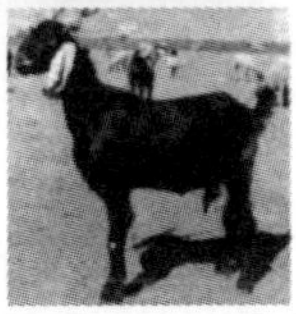

Source: Small Ruminant Rearing Breed Conservation and Genetic Improvement. South Asia pro poor livestock policy programme, a joint initiative of NDDB and FAO, October 2012; http://www.nbagr.res.in/; http://www.icar.org.in/en/node/4684

Chapter 3

LIST OF LESSER KNOWN GOAT GERMPLASM IN INDIA

S.No.	Name	Home Tract	Type
1.	Kodi Adu/Porai Adu	Tamil Nadu	Meat
2.	Salem Black/Karuppu Adu	Tamil Nadu	Meat
3.	Molai Adu	Tamil Nadu	Meat
4.	Pallai Adu /Seeni Adu	Tamil Nadu	Meat
5.	Mahabubnagar/Palamuru	Telangana	Meat
6.	Adilabad Black	Telangana	Meat
7.	Bidri	Karnataka	Meat
8.	Bada Vihana /Dorangi	Odisha	Meat
9.	Dalua/Lenka Chelli	Odisha	Meat
10.	Malkangiri/Koyachelli	Odisha	Meat
11.	Narayanpatna	Odisha	Meat and Milk
12.	Raighari/Nabrangpur	Odisha	Meat
13.	Ghumsari	Odisha	Meat
14.	Kalahandi	Odisha	Meat
15.	Kathewadi	Maharashtra	Meat and milk
16.	Karoli	Rajasthan	Meat
17.	Sojat	Rajasthan	Meat
18.	Battisi	Rajasthan, Uttar Pradesh	Meat and Milk

19.	Bundelkhandi	Uttar Pradesh, Madhya Pradesh	Meat and Milk
20.	Jaunpuri/Jafrabadi	Uttar Pradesh	Milk and Meat
21.	Bareilly	Uttar Pradesh	Meat
22.	Chaugarkha	Uttarakhand	Meat
23.	Udaipuri	Uttarakhand	Meat
24.	Tarai	Uttarakhand	Milk and Meat
25.	Assam Hill	Assam	Meat
26.	Non-pashmina	Jammu and Kashmir	Meat, fiber and milk
27.	Teressa	Andaman and Nicobar Islands	Meat
28.	Local Andaman	Andaman and Nicobar Islands	Meat
29.	Shingarey	Sikkim	Meat

Other lesser known goat germplasm need to be explored

1.	Nagfani	Rajasthan
2.	Patira	Gujarat
3.	Hyderabadi	Andhra Pradesh, Telangana
4.	Totapari	Rajasthan
5.	Kota	Rajasthan

□□□

Chapter 4

DESCRIPTION OF LESSER KNOWN GOAT GERMPLASM

1. KODI ADU/ PORAI ADU

Home Tract: Tamil Nadu

Kodi Adu breed is distributed in south-eastern coastal region of Tamil Nadu. The main breeding tract of this breed is Ottapidram, Pudur and Naglapuram Panchayat unions of Tuticorin district and adjoining areas of Ramanathapuram district besides Puddukottai, Tirunelveli, Tanjore and a part of South Arcot districts (Jain et al., 2000; Tiruvenkadan, 2012). These goats are maintained by landless labourers and marginal farmers in the breeding tract. These goats are also reared along with the sheep flocks by the nomads for leading the migrating flocks which causes the distribution of these goats to other districts. The breeding tract is located at 20 to 60 m above mean sea level with mostly black with red soil in some areas. The climate is hot and humid. The average annual minimum and maximum temperature, relative humidity, rainfall arc 22 and 35°C, 66%, 739 mm in 44 rainy days.

Majority of farmers (about 60%) in the breeding tract houses the goats in both open and close space, 20% in open area and 20% in the closed houses. The goat shed is generally attached to or is a part of owner's dwelling. Housing is particularly needed in rainy season; in other seasons the animals are penned in the open fields. Kids are kept in specially designed enclosures locally known as Koodu which are made from bamboo stalks and palmyrah leaves.

The herds are stationary and are maintained solely on extensive grazing/browsing system except few farmers follow supplementation of bran, cake and gram husk to breeding bucks. Most of the grazing is done on fallow land and on road sides. Stubble grazing in the harvested fields is a common practice. The animals cover about 7-8 km daily during grazing. In this area, community grazing is practiced by mixing 4 to 5 herds which are taken out for grazing with 2-3 farmers/goat herders looking after the herds. Kids are sent for grazing after an age of about 3 months; till that time they are kept at home and fed with sisbania and neem leaves. The major tree species found in this area are babool *(Accacia nilotica)*, umbrella thorn *(Accacia planiforns)* and prosopis *(Prosopis juliflora)*. The major cultivated crops are pearl millet *(Pennisetum typhoides)*, pulses *(Phaseolus mungo, Phaseolus aureus, Vigna unguiculata, Dolichos biflorus, Cajanus cajan and Doliichos lablab)*, chilly *(Capsicum annum)* and coriander *(Coriandrum sativum)* (Jain et al., 2000; Tiruvenkadan, 2012).

I. Phenotypic Characteristics

Color - Kodi Adu goats are grouped into two color varieties, viz. Karum porai (blackish) and Chem porai (reddish brown). Admixture of the two colors including various grades is also seen. However, hair coat is predominantly white with the splashes of black or red color. The dorsal line is dark and the color splashes down on both the sides so that the ventral side is almost white. The extremities including face, ears and legs are generally colored and dark.

Ear - Medium in size, curved forward, slightly drooping but alert

Horn - Open apart slightly as they grow upward, backward and curve down or up sharply at the tip

Back - Back line is almost straight

Barrel - Long and slender

Legs - Thin and long which may be an adaptation to cover long distances during grazing and to keep the barrel high from the ground

Tail - Thin, medium sized

Udder and teats - Small; teats placed laterally

(Jain *et al.*, 2000; Tiruvenkadan, 2012)

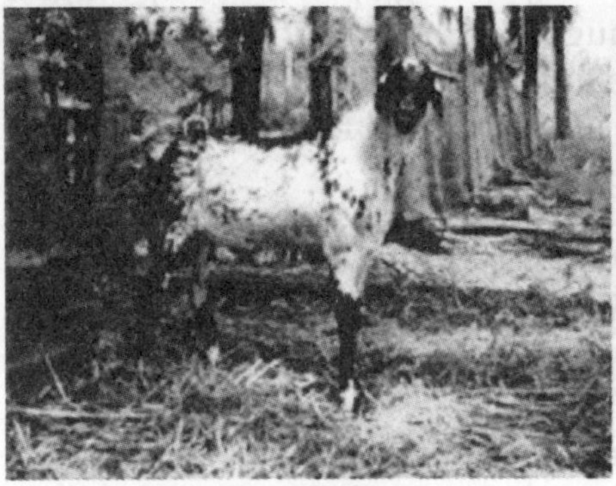	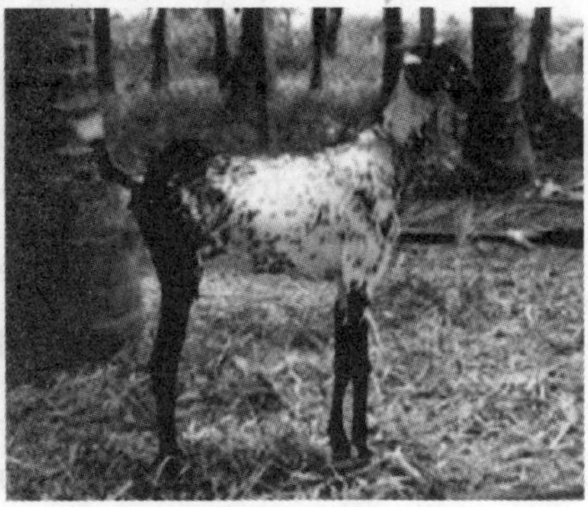
Kodi Adu buck	**Kodi Adu doe**

(Adopted from Tiruvenkadan, 2012)

II. Body measurements (adult goats)

The animals are tall, long, lean and leggy with slender body. Mariadas (1996) also reported that Kodi Adu goats are very tall and their average height is more than Kanni Adu goats.

Traits (cm)	Male	Female
Body length	74.32	72.57
Height at withers	87.07	81.07
Chest girth	82.63	76.96
Horn length	19.0	12.6
Ear length	15.27	
Tail length	17.19	

III. Body weights

Body weight	Male	Female
Adult weight (kg)	39.50	32.17

(Jain *et al.*, 2000)

IV. Reproductive and productive characteristics

The Kodi Adu goat is not seasonal breeders. Kidding occurs round the year however, in January-February, June-July and September-October months, maximum kiddings are observed. There is no systematic selection for breeding males or females. However, male kids are selected for body weight and size based on visual appraisal. Few males are castrated and kept in the flock for sale or religious sacrifice. In general, only male kids are sold between

3-5 months of age @ Rs 500-800 depending upon the body weight. Adult females are sold for slaughter if they are not able to browse or walk. Besides sale of male kids for meat, some income is also generated from the penning in agricultural fields in lieu of land fertility by droppings during the stay.

Traits	Average age (months)/Remarks
Age at first kidding	15-18
Kidding interval	8-10
Multiple births	Primiparous does generally give birth to singles whereas twinning is common in the pluriparous does. Triplets are also seen in a few does depending upon herd size, care taken by the grazer and feed supplementation.
Meat and Milk yield	This goat is mainly reared for meat production. Does are poor in milk production and are not milked for human consumption. Sometimes milk is even not sufficient for kids. Hence milk is exclusively used for suckling by the kids.
Diseases/Mortality/ Health measures	These goats are less susceptible to various diseases and no prophylactic measures are followed for disease control except in case of an outbreak. Anthrax and parasitic infections are major diseases prevalent in the area. For containment of ectoparasitic infestation, hair cutting is practiced and dipping of animals using pesticides is also followed, if needed.

(Jain *et al.*, 2000; Tiruvenkadan, 2012)

2. SALEM BLACK GOATS / KARUPPU ADU

Home Tract: Tamil Nadu

Salem Black goats are distributed in Salem, Dharmapuri, Krishnagiri, Erode, Namakkal and Karur districts of Tamil Nadu (Tiruvenkadan and Karunanithi, 2006). The name 'Salem black' derived from the place in which it is actually originated i.e. Salem district in Tamil Nadu. These goats are tall and predominantly black in colour. The breeding tract of this Salem black goat lies in the north-western agro-climatic zone of Tamil Nadu and the climate is generally hot, semi-arid and tropical in nature. The flock size greatly varies from 2-5 to 50-70, with the majority being 10 to 30 goats, with population of around 86000 goats inhabiting the breeding tract. The percentage of farmers having a flock size of 0-10, 11-20, 21-30, 31-40 and more than 40 was 1.8, 24.6, 43.8, 10.5 and 19.3%, respectively (Tiruvenkadan and Karunanithi, 2006). This goat is mainly reared for meat production. Apart from the phenotypic characterization, the molecular characterization of this goat using microsatellite markers clearly showed that the distribution pattern of alleles and polymorphism in Salem Black goats is similar to the already recognized goat breeds like Kanni Adu, Tellicherry and Barbari which is sufficient enough to qualify for recognition as new goat breeds of India (Thilagam *et al.*, 2011).

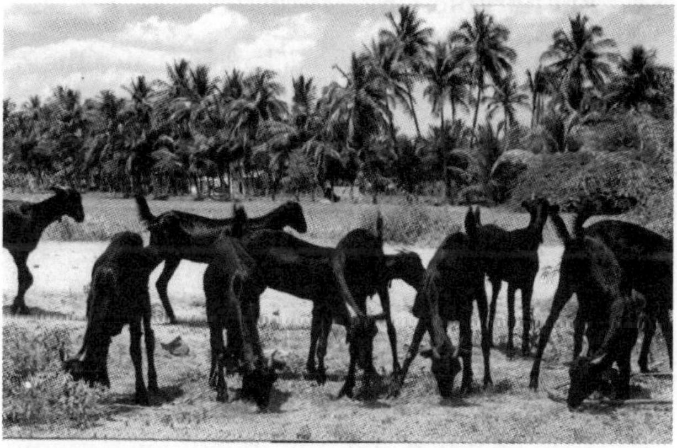

These goats are raised under solely on extensive grazing/ browsing up to a distance of 3-6 km for 7-8 h daily in the bushes along road sides, uncultivable lands, forest areas and harvested fields except 33% flocks are reared under semi intensive system i.e. grazing plus concentrates supplementation. Since these goats are very tall with lengthy body, they consume tree leaves in the forest easily. The main sources of fodder are local weeds on the banks of dry and wet lands, leaves from harvested crops and lopped tree leaves. During the scarcity (summer) of feed/fodder, goats are fed with Acacia pods, tapioca leaves, rind and thippy and dry fodders like groundnut hay, paddy straw and horse gram hay. The kids are not sent for grazing till the completion of after 3 months age in which they are fed with does milk, local weeds, grasses, tree leaves and harvested crops (Tiruvenkadan and Karunanithi, 2006).

Most of the goats (89%) are housed in night hours only after the animals have returned from the grazing fields and are housed with open (75%), half open (12%) and closed type pens (13%), which are well ventilated. The open type enclosure, are made of half walled bamboo sticks having separate shelter for night watchman and kids, are usually placed in the harvested/empty agricultural fields for manure purposes and is shifted to the nearest place daily so as to cover the entire field. Night watchman shelter usually present inside the open type enclosures which serves the purpose of protection of goats from extreme weather and also used as the covered area of the enclosures. Separate shelter for kids is also constructed either inside or near to the open type enclosures using bamboo and palmyra leaves. In half open and closed type sheds also, a small partition is made to accommodate the kids. Mostly the live goats are sold either directly in weekly market (74%) by the farmers or through middlemen and commission agents (26%) (Tiruvenkadan and Karunanithi, 2006).

I. Phenotypic Characteristics

Color - Completely black coat, hence the name black is added as suffix after the *name* of place "Salem" in the breed name. Jain *et al.* (2000) observed white hair coat predominantly with splashes of black or red colour

Head - Straight; medium in length with a medium to broad forehead

Eyelash - Black color

Muzzle - Grey color, tapering

Ear - Leaf like and semi-pendulous, medium to long size

Horn - Ash grey to grey in color with no typical horn pattern

Top line - Almost straight

Flank - Moderate in size and not too wide

Thigh- Lean and not well developed

Legs - Long, lean and straight squarely set under the body

Hooves and dewclaws- Grey in colour

Tail - Thin, medium in length and curled upwards

Udder and teats - Small and round udder, not well developed, tightly attached to the belly with small conical teats placed laterally

(Tiruvenkadan and Karunanithi, 2006)

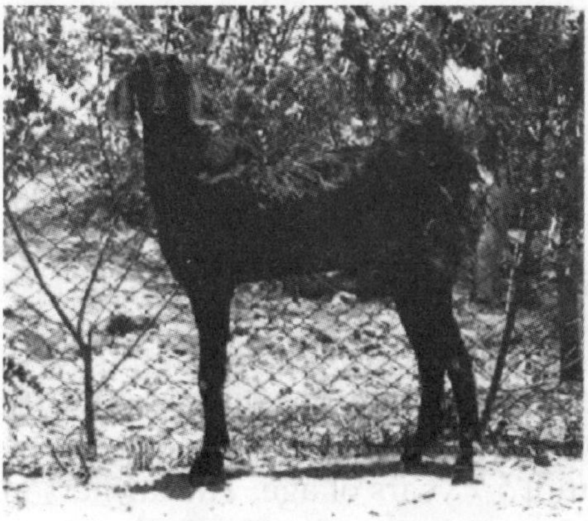

Salem black buck

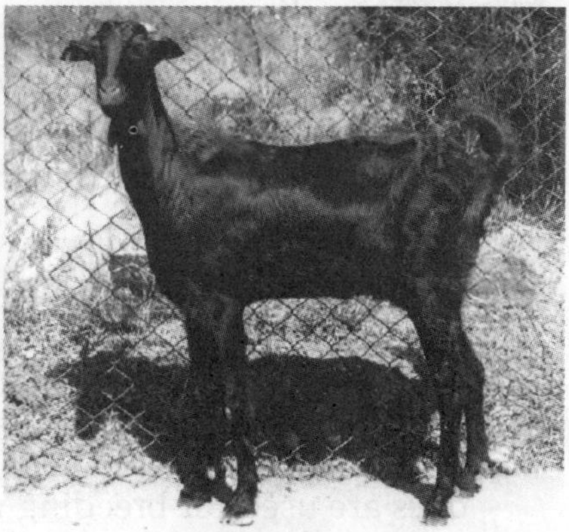

Salem black doe

Courtesy: Personal communication by Dr. Tiruvenkadan

II. Body measurements (adult goats)

Salem Black goats are tall animals with a lean body. Salem Black goats can be grouped under large breeds since its height at withers is more than 65 cm (Devendra and Burns, 1983).

Traits (cm)	Male	Female
Body length	75.0	69.8
Height at withers	86.0	75.5
Chest girth	79.6	73.1
Horn length	20.0	13.7
Ear length	17.2	16.0
Tail length	20.4	17.6

III. Body weights

Average body weight (kg)	Male	Female
Birth weight	2.6	2.4
3 m weight	8.6	8.5
6 m weight	12.1	12.1

9 m weight	14.4	13.9
12 m weight	22.6	18.6
Adult weight - Two tooth	25.8	22.5
Adult weight - Four tooth	28.5	24.7
Adult weight - Six tooth	36.4	26.4
Adult weight - Eight tooth/ full mouth	38.5	29.5

(Tiruvenkadan and Karunanithi, 2006)

IV. Reproductive and productive characteristics

Almost all the male kids and old does are sold for meat purposes and only few young males are selected for breeding at an early age. Bucks are retained for mating up to 5 years of age and the does are used for breeding until 5-7 years of age. The farmers in the breeding tract usually exchange the breeding bucks from one flock to another where only in few flocks (12%); the males are not maintained and are served by bucks of neighbouring flocks on small payment basis. The Salem Black goat seems to have good reproduction potential in terms of early sexual maturity and prolificacy. Most of the females get mated in first oestrus itself due to the presence of bucks all the time in flock with does and the farmers do not have control over mating. Majority (3/4) of does in the flock kidded well before the eruption of the first pair of permanent incisors.

Traits	Average (month; range)/Remarks
Age at first mating in bucks	9.5 (7-12)
Age at first service in nannies	9.7 (6-13)
Age at first kidding	14.8 (11-18)
Kidding interval	7.1 (6-9)
Litter Size	1.6 (1-4)
Litter size (%)	
Single	51.4
Twins	40.0
Triplets	8.2
Quadruplets	0.4
	(Multiple birth: 48.6%)

Meat and Milk yield	These goats are mostly reared for meat; usually does are not milked and kids are allowed to suckle their does till marketing.
Diseases/Mortality/ Health measures	All common goat diseases occur. Vaccination is practiced in case of out breaks. Deworming of the animals is practiced at regular intervals. Salem Black goats are considered as hardy with low overall mortality of 7.5 and 2.3% in kids and adults, respectively which indicate its innate resistance to the harsh climatic conditions prevailing in its original habitat.

(Tiruvenkadan and Karunanithi, 2006)

3. MOLAI ADU

Home Tract: Tamil Nadu

Molai Adu goats are predominantly distributed in Gobichetti-palayam, Bhavani, Sathyamangalam, and Perunthurai Taluks of Erode District and are also found in Namakkal, Salem and Karur Districts in Tamil Nadu (Mariadas, 1996). The flocks are maintained by several communities and are mixed with local goats of different colors. This goat is mainly reared for meat production.

I. Phenotypic Characteristics

Color - Mostly white, sometimes varies from complete white to light brown shades

Ear - Long and drooping

Horn - Does are not horned, that is the reason it is called as 'Molai Adu'

"Molai" means hornless and "Adu" means goat in Tamil language. Bucks are mostly horned, however, 5-10 % doe's possesses horns and few bucks are seen without horns

Legs - Moderate

Tail - Moderate

(Animal Genetic Resources of Tamil Nadu; www.tanuvas.ac.in)

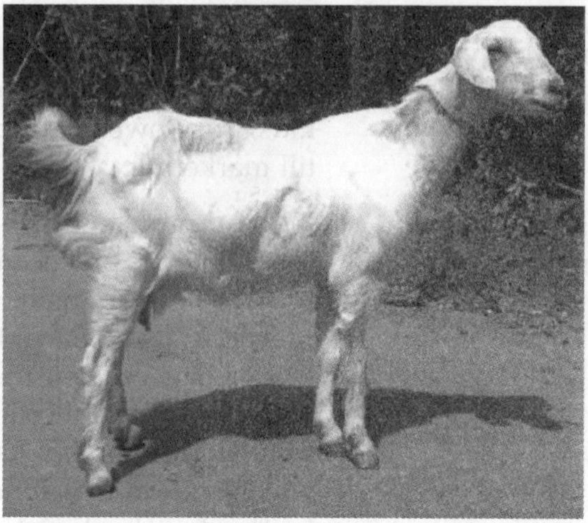

Molai Adu doe

(Adopted from Animal Genetic Resources of Tamil Nadu; www.tanuvas.ac.in)

II. Body measurements (adult goats)

The Molai Adu is moderate in size with musculature. They have compact and low set body.

Traits (cm)	Male	Female
Body length	71.4	69.6
Height at withers	75.4	66.9
Chest girth	75.3	71.8

III. Body weights

Average body weight	Male	Female
Adult weight (kg)	36.42	30.5

4. PALLAI ADU /SEENI ADU

Home Tract: Tamil Nadu

Pallai Adu is one of the indigenous goats distributed in southern parts of Tamil Nadu. Locally the goat is also called as Seeni Adu, because of its promising reproductive performance. Pallai Adu is one of the three indigenous goat breeds distributed in in Karungulam and Ottapidaram blocks of Thoothukudi district and Palayamkottai block of Tirunelveli district of Tamil Nadu (Ravimurugan *et al.*, 2009). Kanni

Adu and Kodi Adu are the other two major indigenous goat breeds found in the Pallai Adu breeding tract (Ravimurugan *et al.*, 2009). The climate of the Pallai Adu breeding tract is generally hot and humid with the ambient temperature ranging from 24.5 to 35.4° C. The maximum precipitation is contributed by the northeast monsoon (551.1 mm) followed by the southwest monsoon (151.1 mm). The soil in the distribution areas is red sandy. The main occupation of the farmers rearing Pallai Adu goat is agriculture (70 %). Pallai Adu is managed exclusively on extensive grazing at all age groups and physiological stages. Mostly goats are kept inside the shelter especially during night hours and the sheds were adjacent to the farmers' house. The mean flock size is 21.2 which ranged from 15 to 35. Pallai Adu is an excellent medium stature food animal and has high litter size, less kidding interval and better adaptability to rural environment, which could increase the overall economics of rural livelihood. This goat is mainly reared for meat production (Ravimurugan *et al.*, 2009).

I. Phenotypic Characteristics

Pallai Adu goats are medium sized short animals with compact body.

Color - Predominantly yellowish brown, few animals have white with mixtures of black or brown colour. Moreover very few animals have black or brown head

Hair- Males have fairly long, straight and rough hairs on neck and withers; Females have short, straight and sleek hairs in almost all parts of the body

Head - Straight

Ear - Medium, leaf like and semi pendulous

Horn - Thick and long; in kids, horn spurs are present

Udder - Fully developed with conical shaped teats

(Ravimurugan *et al.*, 2009)

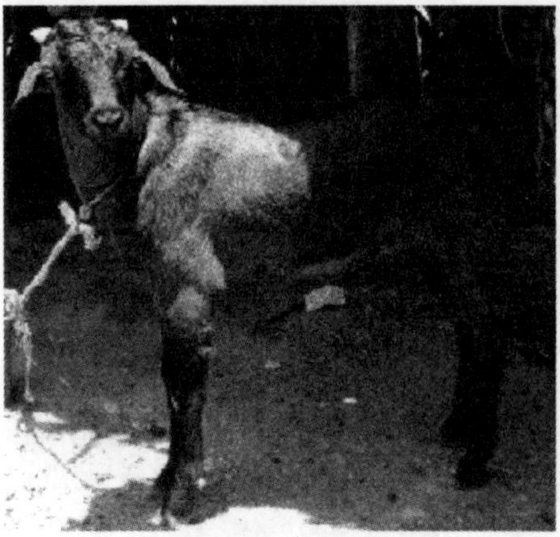

Pallai Adu buck

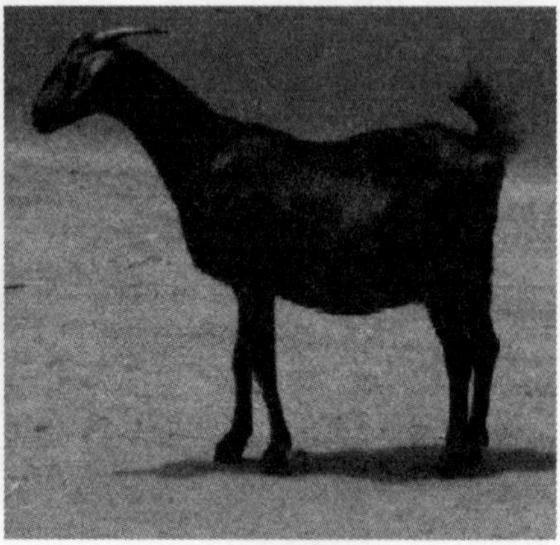

Pallai Adu doe

(Adopted from Mariadas, 1996; Ravimurugan *et al.*, 2009)

II. Body measurements (adult goats) (Ravimurugan *et al.*, 2009)

Traits (cm)	Male	Female
Body length	55.30	50.33
Height at withers	74.34	65.24
Chest girth	70.08	68.05
Horn length	12.75	11.16
Ear length	11.22	11.05
Tail length	15.03	14.84

III. Body weights

Average body weight (kg)	Male	Female
Birth weight	1.85	1.75
Adult weight	21.19	20.25

IV. Reproductive and Productive characteristics

Locally the goat is also called as Seeni Adu, because of its promising reproductive performance (highly prolific) which is better than the Kanni Adu and Kodi Adu, the other two major indigenous goat breeds found in the Pallai Adu breeding tract. The kids born as triplets and quadruplets were found to mature late and also had more age at first kidding, which might be due to their slow growth rate in early days.

Traits	Average age (months)
Age at first mating/sexual maturity in bucks	8.08
Age at first mating/sexual maturity in does	8.45
Age at first kidding	12.84
Kidding interval	7.75
Litter size (%)	
Single	12.1
Twins	75.2
Triplets	10.6
Quadruplets	2.1

(Mariadas, 1996; Ravimurugan *et al.*, 2009)

5. MAHABUBNAGAR/PALAMURU GOATS

Home Tract: Telangana

Mahabubnagar goats are mainly distributed in Gadwal, Mahabubnagar, Nagarkurnool, Narayanpet and Shadnagar divisions of Mahabubnagar district and Chevella division in Ranga Reddy and Deverakonda division in Nalgonda districts of Telengana and is well known for their production potential (Ekambaram *et al.,* 2011a). Goat rearing in this tract appears to be more profitable than sheep due to the ability of goats to thrive on harsh conditions, disease resistance, high prolificacy etc.

The average flock size in the breeding tract is around 44 with majority of farmers maintained 26-50 goats per flock (58%) followed by 51-75 goats per flock (21.3%), 1-25 goats per flock (14.7%), 76-100 goats per flock (4%) and above 100 goats per flock (2%). The goats are mostly reared by landless and marginal farmers on stationary type of keeping and only 2.7% farmers followed either migration system alone or migration with stationary type. Goats are reared mostly on extensive system of rearing (72%) with rest in semi intensive and 0.67% under intensive rearing system. The preference of extensive rearing system with more than 7-8 hrs grazing covering 6-10 km daily by the farmers in the forests, waste and community lands is mainly due to the abundant availability of browsing materials, cropping, pastures etc during different seasons. The goats under semi intensive system are usually supplemented with concentrates, crop by-products, etc after returning from grazing especially during lean periods under group feeding conditions. These goats has liking for a wide variety of feeds. The watering facility for goats are provided by the farmers both at sheds and grazing fields and few farmers (26%) did not give water in sheds (Ekambaram *et al.*, 2011b).

The independent shelters for goats are constructed by 63.51% of farmers with rest constructed the goat shelters as part of their houses to safe guard the animals during night time. Majority of farmers (94.7%) in the breeding tract houses the goats during night time to protect them from the wild animals and thefts, whereas 2% farmers houses during day time. The farmers provide both closed (60%) and open (40%) type of houses for their goats. The closed houses are constructed with walls made of locally available materials and fences made of wooden or stone poles or thorny bushes whereas, goats under open houses are kept under trees, open areas, foot hills etc. The *kutcha* type of floors in goat houses are mostly preferred by farmers and are prepared economically with locally available *morram* and gravel as this materials maintains coolness in summer, warmness during winter and quickly absorbs the moisture resulting from urine, defecations etc. The thatched roof, made of locally available materials like paddy straw, *tunga*, maize and *jowar* straws, forest tree leaves, bushes etc, was preferred for goat houses by 52.7% farmers followed by asbestos roof (18.2%) and roof made of tiles, iron and plastic sheets, polyethylene covers and cement roofs (29.1%) (Ekambaram *et al.,* 2011b).

Most of the farmers (71.3%) usually disposes kids at an early age of 4-6 months indirectly complementing the weaning process in villages and did not follow practice of weaning in goat flock, 15.3% marketed before weaning (3 m), 9.3% marketed between 7 -10 months of age and only 4% farmers marketed their goats at optimum age of 11-13 months for getting remunerative price as well as to produce tender chevon. Farmers dispose off their animals to the only available market channel *i.e.* butcher after prolonged bargaining and usually sell in their own villages (52.7%) followed by near-by livestock shandy (23.3%) and 24% farmers sell their animals at both places. Mostly farmers sell their goats based on the size of the animal and discretion of the butcher (65.3%) followed by size or shape of the animal (26.7%), discretion of the butcher (2.7%) and merely 2% farmers sell their goats on live weight basis (Ekambaram *et al.,* 2011b).

I. Phenotypic Characteristics

These goats are comparable with most of the native breeds of goats in morphological characters.

Color - Predominantly bicolor (63.5%) with the admixture of black and white (30.9%), brown and white (22.1%) and black and brown (10.4%). Apart from bicolor coat, these goats have single (25%) and multi-color patterns (11.5%). The single color animal categories represent black (9.69%), brown (9.06%) and white (6.2%). The apparent wide variation in coat color among Mahabubnagar goats observed is indicative of the fact that it has not yet been purified through selective breeding and therefore great opportunities exist for its improvement.

Head - Straight (74.3%), slightly convex (21.0%) and convex (4.7)

Ear - Mostly pendulous (91.6%) followed by erect (4.6%) and horizontal (3.8%)

Horn - 57% goats have straight horns with remaining proportion having curved horns with mostly oriented backward (46.2%), backward and downward (40.3%). The horns are mostly medium sized (15–25 cm length, 63.5%) followed by Small (less than 15 cm, 25.7%) and large sized ones (more than25 cm, 10.8%)

Beard - Majority of goats have beard (86.0%)

Wattles - Present only in 34.3% of goats

(Ekambaram *et al.*, 2011a)

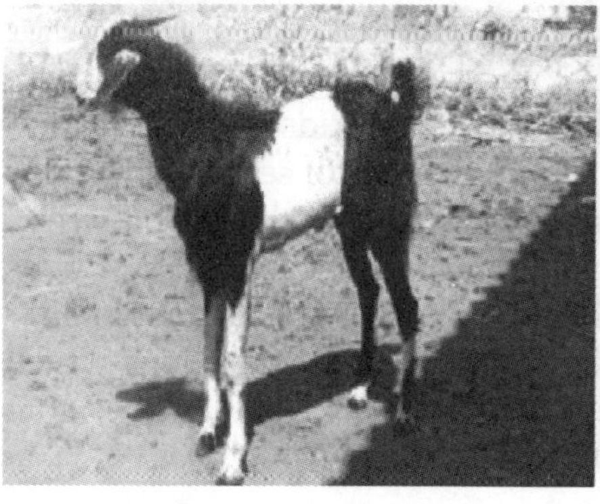

Mahabubnagar buck

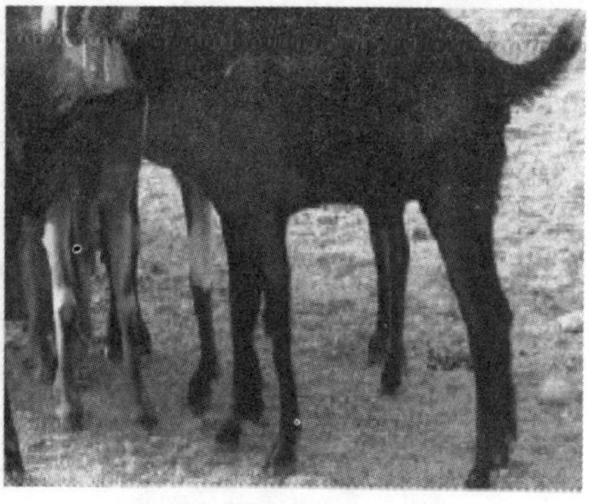

Mahabubnagar doe

(Adopted from Ekambaram *et al.*, 2011a)

II. Body weights

Average body weight (kg)	Male	Female
Birth weight	2.16	2.11
3 m weight	9.03	8.37
6 m weight	12.77	11.69
9 m weight	15.66	14.37
12 m weight	18.81	16.97

(Ekambaram *et al.*, 2011a)

III. Reproductive and productive characteristics

The farmers in the breeding tract do not follow any selection for breeding males and except following conventional approaches like good physical appearance and body size, timely culling of unproductive animals, animals with stunted growth and deformities etc which is complementing the selection of goats as well. Mostly bucks are allowed along with females in a flock throughout the year which takes care of heat detection as well as natural mating. No castration is followed in males for getting higher body weights during growth phase. The male: female ratio is usually maintained at optimum level of 1:20-30 in the flocks which might be helping in obtaining higher kidding percentage, lower kid mortality due to reproductive problems and maintenance of genetic distance among progeny. Only 25% farmers in the breeding tract follows the rotation of their breeding bucks by means of exchange, replacement etc for avoiding inbreeding, getting higher reproductive rate and body weights at various ages in the flock. The average litter size is 1.89 ± 0.02 which ranged from 1.77 to 2.07 and twinning constituted more than fifty percent of the multiple births. Six kids were born from does in 0.23 per cent of kidding and one case of septuplets which is a rare phenomenon in the field of small ruminant reproduction. The incidence of multiple births increases as the parity of does increased indicating the highly prolific nature of Mahabubnagar goats and efficient reproducibility under field conditions which are comparable with those of some of established Indian goat breeds (Ekambaram *et al.,* 2011c).

Traits	Average age/ Remarks
Age at first mating (days)	304.87
Age at first kidding (days)	455.65
Kidding interval (days)	254.92
Litter size (%)	
Single	30.08
Twins	51.45
Triplets	15.95
Quadruplets	2.29
Hexaplets	0.23
Meat yield (farm bred, 1 year age)	
Pre slaughter weight (kg)	24.36
Empty body weight (kg)	18.29
Hot carcass weight (kg)	10.90
Dressing % (on PSW)	44.60
Dressing % (on EBW)	59.74
Diseases/Mortality/ Health measures	All common goat diseases occur. Mostly the flock mortality occurs with normal range of 6-10% except 11-15% occurs in few flocks. The prevalence of pneumonia condition and contagious ecthyma were very high in field conditions, and followed by PPR and FMD. Due to lack of housing facility, the animals were exposed to extreme weather conditions which resulted in pneumonia and ecthyma conditions. Majority of the (82.1%) farmers practices de-worming twice a year, 11.32% practices once and 6.6% thrice a year. The prescribed ectoparasitic control measures and vaccination schedules were

not practiced by 90% of the farmers due to lack of awareness and misconception among farmers particularly shepherds. However farmers are well aware of using veterinary dispensary or hospital services for treatment of the diseased goats. Majority of the farmers did not know the significance of proper disposal of dead animals and the mode of spread of infectious diseases from one out break to other places and disposes dead animals in open fields, on road sides etc.

(Ekambaram *et al.*, 2010, 2011c)

6. ADILABAD BLACK

Home Tract: Telangana

Adilabad goats are mainly distributed in Inder valley and Khannapur mandals of Adilabad district of Telangana (Raja *et al.*, 2011). This district is one of the poorest districts of the Andrapradesh state before partition having 2.1 million people living in 1613 square km with 44% forest degraded land. These goats are mainly reared by 'Gonds' tribes under extensive system/zero input system. Goats are generally grazed in the forest lands from 8.00 AM to 6.00 PM in the day time and during night, 5-6 farmers collective keep their goats outside the village (Raja *et al.*, 2011).

I. Phenotypic characteristics

Color – Body coat is black with white patches on the ears.

II. Body measurements (adult goats)

Traits (cm)	Male	Female
Body length	64.19	64.06
Height at withers	80.08	77.23
Chest girth	77.59	76.29
Paunch girth	77.97	78.30

Horn length	13.63	12.49
Ear length	16.44	15.80
Tail length	15.80	13.28

III. Body weights

Average body weight (kg)	Male	Female
Birth weight	2.00	-
0-3 m weight	9.15	-
4-6 m weight	14.26	-
7-12 m weight	17.28	-
Adult weight	34.28	31.98

(Raja *et al.*, 2011)

7. BIDRI

Place of origin: Karnataka

Bidri goats are distributed mainly in Bidar District of Karnataka State.

I. Phenotypic characteristics

Color - Predominantly black coat (54.75%) followed by admixture of black and white (30.20), black and brown (15.05%). Similarly majority of goats have black skin (44.77%) followed by white (30.04%), grey (22.04%), pink (2.72%) and brown (0.43%) color skin. The majority of blackness of skin and coat is due to the contribution of Osmanabadi genes towards Bidri gene pool. Muzzle and eyelids (more than80%), hoof (71%), horn (63%) are also black in color.

Forehead - Mostly straight (98%) with few concave (0.37%) and convex (1.71%) shape

Ear - Mostly pendulous (94.98%), horizontal (3.31%) and erect (1.71%)

Horn - 77.11% goats have horns with straight (22.35%) and curved (60.83%)

Beard - Few goats have beard (5%)

Wattles - Present only in 2% of goats

Tail- Mostly medium in length (84%) with remaining goats as short tailed

(Shettar and Rudresh, 2003a)

II. Body measurements (adult goats)

Traits (cm)	Pooled across sexes
Body length	40.18
Height at withers	70.69
Chest girth	72.38
Ear length	15.36

III. Body weights

Average body weight (kg)	Pooled across sexes
Birth -1 m weight	5.69
1-3 m weight	9.62
3-6 m weight	16.53
6-12 m weight	23.42
More than12 m weight	31.23

(Shettar and Rudresh, 2003b)

8. BADA VIHANA/DORANGI

Home Tract: Odisha

Bada Vihana goats are distributed mostly in Nayagarh district and southern parts of Khurda district of Odisha (Kornel *et al.*, 2006). This breed has been developed by the farmers in its breeding tract by crossing Ganjam bucks and Black Bengal does for last two-three decades and subsequently inter-breeding of crossbreds coupled with selection. This crossing practice is continuing and the resultant crossbred individuals constantly infused in to this breed. The flock size greatly varies from 5-30 with 1-2 breeding bucks. These goats are raised under small holder production systems having crop and goat production as an integrated component. Goats are exclusively managed under extensive grazing along with cattle and sheep. Sometimes, goats are grazed separately in nearby forests and fallow lands after mixing many flocks by a hired labor appointed jointly by the flock owners (Kornel *et al.*, 2006). Almost all the farmers provide either pucca or kutcha shelter in night hours after grazing which protects goats from predation and extreme weather. Shelters are made of locally available materials like wood, bamboo, mud etc. depends on the income of the farmers. Kids are not weaned and continue to suckle their mothers till nest kidding and kids are allowed for grazing with does after 2 months of age. Majority of farmers provide common salt lick for their goats fortnightly and no other supplementation is provided. These goats drink water in the grazing fields if available else drinking water is made available at enclosures. The animals of this breed are well adapted to their habitat and can survive scarcity of feed and are fairly resistant to internal parasites. They are relatively more resistant against most of the common goat diseases compared to Ganjam and Black Bengal goats (Kornel *et al.,* 2006).

I. Phenotypic characteristics

Color - Coat color varies widely; black, brown, mixed black and brown with some white patches. It is also known as 'Dorangi goats' in Nayagarh due to its bicolor coat or nature of its two breed cross

Hair- Usually short; long hairs are present in neck, tail and thigh region

Head - Straight with slight convexity in the middle above nasal septum; larger in males than females

Ear - Mostly drooping except in few cases, it is horizontal or straight; medium to large size

Horn - Small horns usually straight and extends angularly upward and sideward; long horns are curved inward and present mostly in male

Beard - Present in less than 5% of animals

Wattles- Present in about 10% of animals

Tail - Small and thin

Udder and teats- Small to medium

(Kornel *et al.,* 2006)

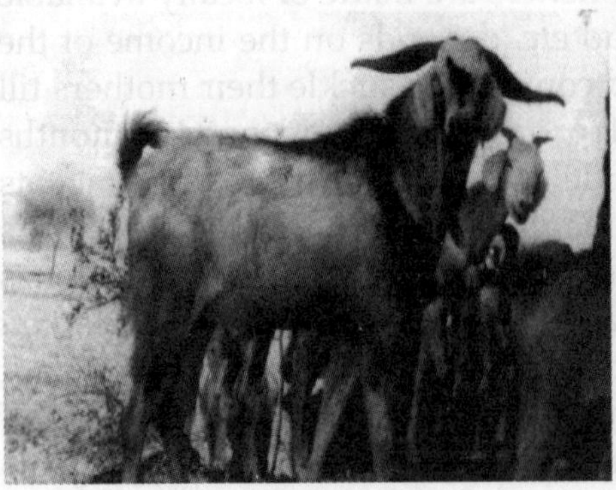

Bada Vihana buck

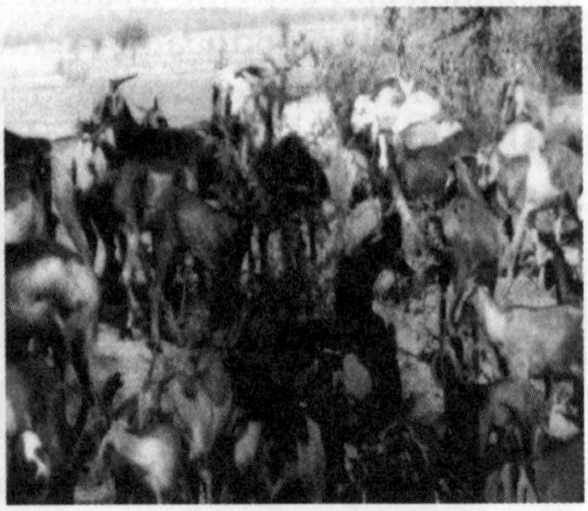

Bada Vihana doe

(Adopted from Kornel *et al.*, 2006)

II. Body measurements (adult goats) (Kornel *et al.*, 2006)

The Bada Vihana goat is medium sized prolific breed and is larger than Black Bengal and smaller than Ganjam goats.

Traits (cm)	Male	Female
Body length (L1)	52	49.2
Body length (L2)	58	57.1
Height at withers	67.2	64.7
Chest girth or circumference	67.7	65.8
Paunch girth or Abdomen girth	74.7	80.2
Neck girth	37.7	33.7
Thigh girth	39.2	34.5
Head length	25.7	19.9
Horn length	17.2	11.4
Ear length	13.2	13.3
Tail length	14.3	13.3

(L1: point of wither to hip joint; L2: hip joint to shoulder joint)

III. Body weights

Average body weight	Male	Female
Adult weight (kg)	27.0	24.4

IV. Reproductive and productive characteristics

Bucks are selected based on their phenotypic traits, vigor and size. Usually no selection is practiced in does and all are used for breeding except those in poor body condition or unable to reproduce. The male: female ratio is usually maintained at 1:20 to 1:30 in the flocks. Young bucks are preferred for random mating than older bucks and the use of more than 3 years old bucks are very rare in the flock. There is no exchange of bucks between flocks except in small flocks, where the breeding bucks are brought in to the flock from other flocks on small payment basis. The surplus males which are not required for breeding are castrated and sold at good price due to free of goaty odour.

Traits	Mean age / Remarks
Age at first heat/estrous (months)	12-15
Mean age at first kidding (months)	18
Kidding interval (months)	8.0 (3 kidding in two years)
Incidence of multiple births	
Twins (%)	60
Meat and Milk yield	These goats are mostly reared for meat by self-help groups due to its large body size and higher meat yield. Manure and skin are also of high economic value; usually does are not milked since milk is just enough for kids and kids continue to suckle their mothers till next kidding.
Diseases/Mortality/ Health measures	All common goat diseases occur. Vaccination is practiced regularly except non availability of PPR vaccines cause heavy mortality. These goats are well adapted to their habitat; easily survive with feed scarcity, fairly resistant to gastro intestinal parasites and even more resistant to most of the common goat diseases than Ganjam and Black Bengal goats.

(Kornel *et al.*, 2006)

9. DALUA/LENKA CHELLI

Home Tract: Odisha

Kornel *et al.* (2006) reported that Dalua goats are distributed in Chilika coast of Rambha and Khallikote blocks of Ganjam districts of Odisha and are primarily reared by Golla community in the breeding tract. The local language, 'Dala' means branch and these goats usually feed on branches of trees present in Chilika lake hence the name "Dalua". Though the origin of this breed is not known clearly, it may have been evolved through Ganjam breed since both are having lot of similarities in terms of physical and performance traits. The flock size greatly varies from 20-200 with population of around 20,000 inhabiting the coast of Chilika lake. These goats are raised under small holder production systems solely on extensive grazing either separately or with sheep. Majority of farmers provide common salt lick for their goats monthly and no other supplementation is provided. These goats drink water in the grazing fields in ponds/rivers/streams and no drinking facility is made available in enclosures. Just to reduce the cost of rearing, goats are grazed usually by mixing many flocks by a hired labor appointed jointly by the flock owners. Presently, they pay Rs. 1000 per month for 200 goats. Flocks are semi-nomadic type and move from place to place in search of browsing materials near the house of owner and are housed there itself in open enclosures throughout the year, unlike Ganjam goats which are mostly kept in fields away from farmers home. Kids are not weaned and continue to suckle their mothers till next kidding in the morning and evening. These goats are of special significance to Golla community as they primarily depend on sheep and goats for their livelihood by sale, gift and sacrifice live animals, sale of ghee and manure. The marketing of ghee is done by women while sale of live animals is carried by men (Kornel *et al.,* 2006).

I. Phenotypic characteristics

Color - Predominantly black coat (90%), remaining 10% is brown, mixture of black and brown; the luster and intensity of black or brown varies individually, although the frequency of jet black and dark brown coat is more than light color

Hair- Usually short, lustrous and black in black color coat or brown, mixture of black and brown in other cases. Hairs in tail are longer than body and few goats have long hairs in thigh region. Males have slightly longer hairs than females and are seen in all parts of body

Head - Generally straight or slight convex and color is same as of body

Ear - Fairly large and slightly drooping

Horn - Usually big horns extends backward and upward, some cases semi curved; farmers like long horns and give importance for the same at selection

Beard - Absent

Wattles- Mostly absent

Legs - Long legs and placed well apart from each other

Tail - Medium and thin

Udder and teats- Usually small; few goats have medium size

(Kornel *et al.*, 2006)

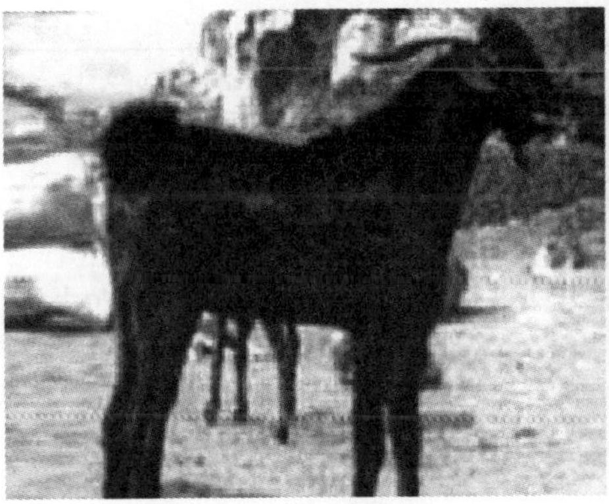

Dalua buck

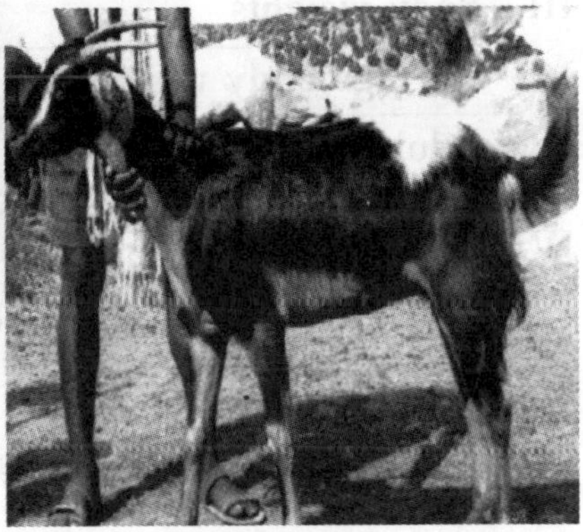

Dalua doe

(Adopted from Kornel *et al.*, 2006)

II. Body measurements (adult goats)

The size of Dalua goats is as tall as Ganjam goats and heavier and taller than Bada Vihana goats.

Traits (cm)	Male	Female
Body length (L1)	54	53.3
Body length (L2)	61.2	60.9
Height at withers	75.5	76.0
Chest girth or circumference	79.0	78.3
Paunch girth or Abdomen girth	85.5	83.8
Neck girth	47.5	40.0
Thigh girth	53.5	39.5
Head length	24.0	21.3
Horn length	27.0	21.2
Ear length	11.5	
(Range: 10.0-13.0)	13.5	
(Range: 12.0-15.0)		
Tail length	13.5	15.8

(L1: point of wither to hip joint; L2: hip joint to shoulder joint)

III. Body weights

Average body weight	Male	Female
Adult weight (kg)	41.0	35.7

IV. Reproductive and productive characteristics

Usually young bucks at the age of 2-3 years are used for breeding purposes at random. Every two years, exchange of bucks between flocks is made to reduce effect of 'inbreeding'. Young bucks are preferred for random mating than older bucks and the use of more than 3 years old bucks are very rare in the flock. There are two breeding seasons viz., September-October and March- April. The first breeding season is not preferred by farmers as kids born during March-April have lower weight gain due to less feed availability and high mortality due to monsoon rains. The male: female ratio is usually maintained at 1:20 to 1:25 in the flocks. The surplus males which are not required for breeding are disposed of at around 12 months and are not castrated. Due to this reason, the meat and milk from Dalua goats give goaty odour similar to Ganjam goats unlike Bada Vihana goats which is free of this bad odour.

Traits	Average age (months)/Remarks
Age at first mating in bucks	12
Age at first heat/estrous	24
Mean age at first kidding	27-30
Kidding interval	12.0 (in 20% goats, 3 kiddings in 2 years)
Litter size (%)	
Single	90
Twins	Very rare
Average milk yield (kg)	0.3-0.5
	Usually does are not milked since milk is just enough for kids and kids continue to suckle their mothers till next kidding. Few farmers milk the does and provide alternate feed to kids; if kids die, then does are milked for preparing 'ghee only' and consumed by them.
Average lactation length (months)	5.0
Diseases/Mortality/ Health measures	All common goat diseases occur. Kid and adult mortality (20% each) includes death from diseases as well as predation and theft; Golla people use indigenous medicines besides worshipping goddesses due to illiteracy and lack of awareness. The non-availability of vaccines and medicines causes heavy mortality in flocks.

(Kornel *et al.*, 2006)

10. MALKANGIRI/KOYACHELLI GOATS

Home Tract: Odisha

Malkangiri goats are distributed in Malkangiri hill districts of Odisha which having 90% forest land (Kornel *et al.*, 2006). Malkangiri goats are medium in size and weight and are reared for meat only. Goats also used for sacrifice and on several occasions as gift resulting in increase of female population. The flock size greatly varies from 7-150 with population of around 50,000 inhabiting the breeding tract however, Verma *et al.* (2013) reported lower flock size of 5-35 in the study area. These goats are raised under small holder production systems having crop and other livestock species like cattle, sheep and poultry as an integrated component. Mostly, these goats are reared on semi- extensive management system. When the goat population is small in the village, these goats usually go for extensive grazing along with cattle and sheep else they are reared and grazed separately in flocks. If flock size is small, they are housed mostly in the house of the owner in a separate space on raised wooden/bamboo floor and the flock size is large, they are reared on open spaces having enclosures throughout the year like Ganjam goats. No supplementation is provided for these goats as they are solely on extensive grazing except kids, apart from milk and not allowed for grazing, they are being given locally available succulent green fodders liked by them. Kids are not weaned and continue to suckle their mothers till next kidding in the morning and evening hours when does are in shed. Just to reduce the cost of rearing, goats are grazed usually by mixing many flocks jointly by the flock owners. Flocks move from place to place in search of browsing materials near the house of owner in the village and most of the flocks reared near forest areas for easy availability of plants and trees for browsing. Since 90% area is forest type, predation from wild animals and wetness of floor is common so the above mentioned type of raised floor sheds is used for protection of goats. In summer, goats are allowed freely in forests to graze after 11 AM after collection of Mahua flowers and goats use to return home themselves from forest. These goats drink water in the grazing fields in ponds/rivers/streams depending on the availability (Kornel *et al.*, 2006).

I. Phenotypic characteristics

Malkangiri goats are taller and heavier than Black Bengal goats but shorter and lighter than Ganjam goats.

Color - Predominantly brown coat (70%), black (25%), white (3%) remaining 2% is mixture of brown, black and white. The face has strips of white or light brown colour extending from base of ear to nose in brown goats. The top line is black. In males black ring is present around the neck. Muzzle and hooves are generally black

Hair - Usually short, Hairs in neck and pubic region are longer, not shorn for hair yield

Head - Generally straight and medium in size

Ear - Erect, medium in size, extend horizontally; rarely pendulous

Horn - Usually straight somewhat flat and extends backward and upward making an acute angle with head. The length and diameter of horns increases with age like other measurable traits till four permanent teeth stage is reached

Beard - Present in 5% goats

Wattles - Present in few goats and small in size

Udder and teats - Usually medium size and round shape

(Kornel *et al.*, 2006)

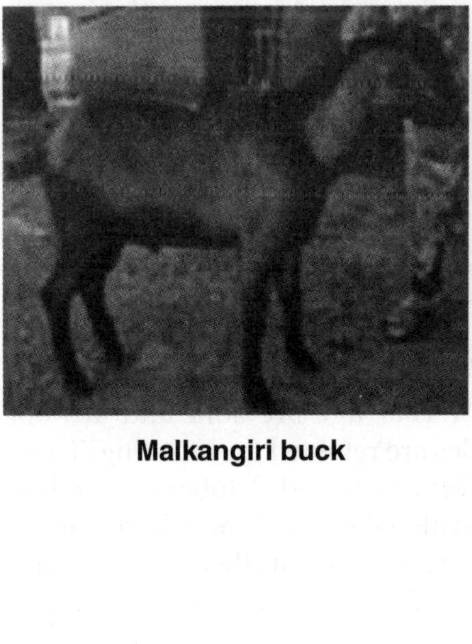

Malkangiri buck

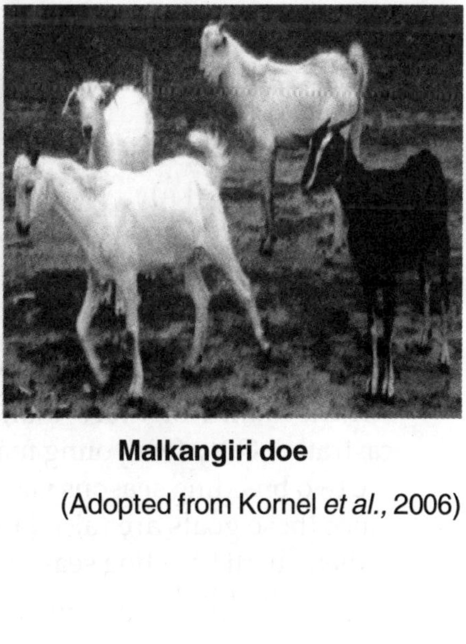

Malkangiri doe

(Adopted from Kornel *et al.*, 2006)

II. Body measurements (adult goats)

Traits (cm)	Male	Female
Body length (L1)	51.6	48.9
Body length (L2)	58.8	56.5
Height at withers	68.2	63.5
Chest girth or circumference	76.2	70.7
Paunch girth or abdomen girth	90.8	83.7
Neck girth	40.0	35.3
Thigh girth	25.0	28.0
Head length	18.6	16.8
Horn length	14.6	12.1
Ear length	11.4	13.5
Tail length	13.4	11.5

(L1: point of wither to hip joint; L2: hip joint to shoulder joint) (Kornel *et al.*, 2006)

III. Body weights (kg)

Average body weight	Male	Female
3m wt	9.00	8.14
6m wt	12.25	11.13
9m wt	14.5	13.20
12m wt	16.67	16.30
Adult weight (kg)	26.73	23.93
Adult weight (kg)		
Kornel *et al.*, 2006	30.2	26.9

(Verma *et al.*, 2015)

IV. Reproductive and productive characteristics

All the males of more than 1 year age are sold and are not castrated. Only few young males are retained for breeding. There are two breeding seasons viz., May-June and October-November. Since these goats are raised mostly near forests and feed scarcity is there, both breeding seasons are preferred as there no difference in growth of kids. The male: female ratio varied from 1:5 to 1:20 in the flocks.

Traits	Average values/ Remarks
Age at first mating in bucks (months)	Less than 12
Age at first heat/estrous (months)	6-7
Mean age at first kidding (months)	12
Kidding interval (months) (2 kiddings in a year)	6
Litter size (%)	
Single (common in first kidders)	15
Twins	80
Triplets	5
Average milk yield (kg)	0.5-0.8 Usually does are not milked since milk is just enough for kids.
Average lactation length (months)	4
Diseases/Mortality/ Health measures	All common goat diseases occur. Kid and adult mortality (20% each) includes death from diseases and predation & theft; Vaccination and deworming is not practiced. Local farmers use indigenous medicines besides worshipping goddesses due to illiteracy and lack of awareness. The non-availability of vaccines and medicines causes heavy mortality in flocks. These goats are well adapted to high temperature and heavy rains their habitat, fairly resistant to most of the common goat diseases including gastro intestinal parasites.

(Kornel *et al.*, 2006; Verma *et al.*, 2015)

11. NARAYANPATNA GOATS

Home Tract: Odisha

Kornel *et al.* (2006) reported that Narayanpatna goats are distributed in Narayanpatna taluk of Koaraput districts of Odisha and reared by Kondh tribes living in the breeding tract. This goat is mainly reared for both for meat due to its large body size and milk due its high milk production (dual purpose) besides for sacrifice and on several occasions as gift with few surplus goats are sold in the market. This breed has been probably evolved by the Kondh tribes through inter breeding of crosses of goats of Odisha and neighboring Andhra Pradesh over time. The flock size greatly varies from 5-100 with population of around 20,000 inhabiting the breeding tract. The management followed by Kondh tribes for these goats are almost similar to rearing practices of Malkangiri goats. Verma *et al.,* (2015) also reported that these goats are reared by Kondhs tribes for meat purposes under extensive rearing with the flock size of 2 to 34.

I. Phenotypic characteristics

Color - Predominantly dull white and dull black (80%); rest is either brown or mixture of black and white and even mixed colour animals are also seen

Hair - Usually short and not shorn for hair yield. Tail hairs are longer than body hairs, thigh hairs are longer and dense

Head - Slightly convex; length of horns increases with age

Ear - Usually erect, few goats pendulous have pendulous type

Horn - Usually small and straight extending either upward and backward or horizontally upward. Length of horns increases with age of goats

Beard - Absent

Wattles - Present in few goats and smaller than in Ganjam goats

Legs - Medium legs, straight and placed well apart from each other

Tail - Medium and thin with long hairs; few farmers clip after kidding to prevent infection. Length of tail increases with age of goats

Udder and teats - Usually medium size; some udders are funnel type with long fall teats

(Kornel *et al.*, 2006)

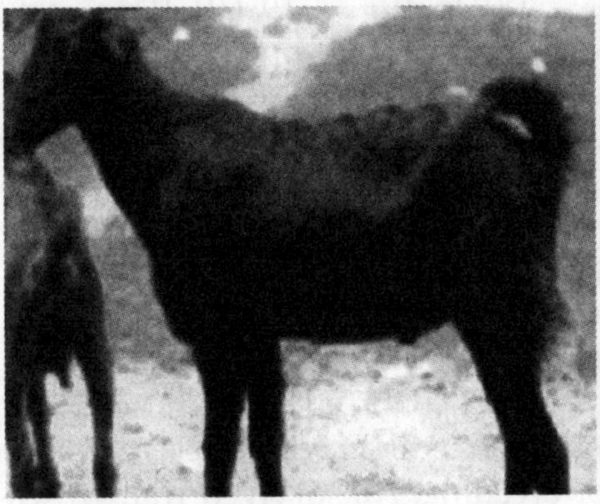

Narayanpatna buck

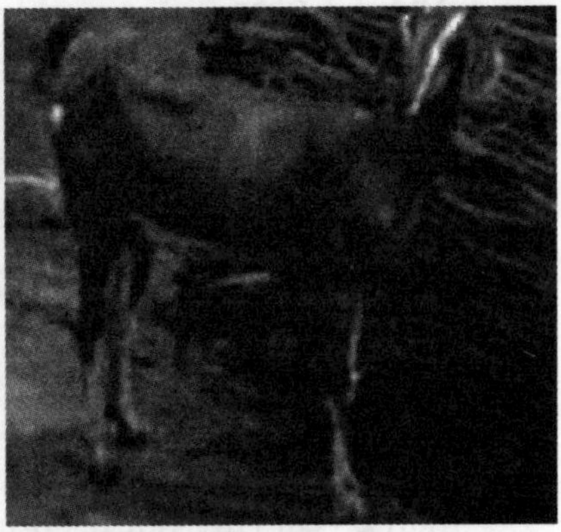

Narayanpatna doe

(Adopted from Kornel *et al.*, 2006)

II. Body measurements (adult goats)

Narayanpatna goats are medium in size, usually bigger than Black Bengal goats but slightly smaller than Ganjam goats.

Traits (cm)	Male	Female
Body length (L1)	56.5	52.3
Body length (L2)	64.5	60.0
Height at withers	77.0	70.0
Chest girth or circumference	88.0	73.4
Paunch girth or abdomen girth	93.5	81.2
Neck girth	47.0	37.3
Thigh girth	41.0	31.6
Head length	18.5	17.1
Horn length	22.5	13.1
Ear length	15.0	14.0
Tail length	15.5	13.7

(L1: point of wither to hip joint; L2: hip joint to shoulder joint)
(Kornel *et al.*, 2006)

III. Body Weights

Average body weight (kg)	Male (range)	Female (range)
About 1 year	18 (16-19)	19 (19-21)
2 permanent teeth	22 (20-24)	20 (19-22)
Adult weight (4-8 teeth)	38 (37-39)	28 (24-36)

IV. Reproductive and productive characteristics

All the males of more than 1 year age are sold and are not castrated. However, flock does not emit goaty odor due to its wider male: female ratio and few farmers do not rear males and borrow male from neighbouring flock for breeding purposes. Only few young males are retained for breeding and bucks aged more than 2 years are not used for breeding. All survived well grown female kids are used for breeding. There are two breeding seasons viz., May- June and October-November Since goats these goats are raised mostly near forests and feed scarcity is there, both breeding seasons are preferred as there no difference in growth of kids. The male: female ratio is 1:20 in the flocks.

Traits	Average age / Remarks
Age at first mating in bucks (months)	Less than 12
Age at first heat/estrous (months)	6-7
Mean age at first kidding (months)	12
Kidding interval (months)	6-7
	(Usually 3 kidding in 2 year)
Litter size (%)	
Single (common in first kidders)	
Twins	80
Triplets	20
Extremely rare	
Average milk yield (kg)	0.6-0.7
	Usually does are not milked since milk is just enough for kids and kids continue to suckle their mothers till next kidding. Few

	farmers milk the does when kids attains 3 months age and provide alternate supplementary feed to kids
Average lactation length (months)	5
Diseases/Mortality/ Health measures	Similar to Malkangiri goats

(Kornel *et al.*, 2006)

12. RAIGHARI/NABRANGPUR GOATS

Home Tract: Odisha

Raighar goats are widely distributed in villages of Raighar, Umerkot and Dabugon blocks of Koraput district and adjacent areas in Nabarangpur district of Odisha (Kornel *et al.,* 2006). This goat is mainly reared for meat and the Gonda and Bhatra tribes of Koraput are the original breeders of these goats. The Raigarhi Goats are popular meat animals in Odisha and are well known for their high prolificacy with frequent twinning and triplet kidding except first kidding which is usually single type.

The flock size greatly varies from very few to 200 with population of around more than 30,000 inhabiting the breeding tract. These goats are raised under small holder production systems having crop and other livestock species like cattle, sheep and poultry as an integrated component. When the goat population is small in the village, these goats usually go for extensive grazing along with cattle and sheep else they are reared and grazed separately in flocks. The management practices followed for this goat also similar to rearing practices of Malkangiri goats (Kornel *et al.,* 2006).

I. Phenotypic characteristics

Raigari goats, reared mainly for meat, are medium in size. These goats have distinct morphological features, different from those of Ganjam, Bengal and Malkangiri goats available in Odisha.

Color - Predominantly solid brown (60%), black (30%) or mixture of black and brown (10%) and without any patchy pattern. white stripes on both sides extending from the forehead up to the nose is a constant feature. White or light brown colour strips extending from base of the ear to muzzle are present on either side of the nose line. Muzzle colour is black or brown and hooves are black or grey

Hair – Usually short, long hairs in tail, thigh and neck than body

Head - Straight

Ear - Usually erect and extend horizontally

Beard - Absent

Wattles- Absent

Udder and teats- Usually medium size, well developed with medium sized teats

(Kornel *et al.*, 2006)

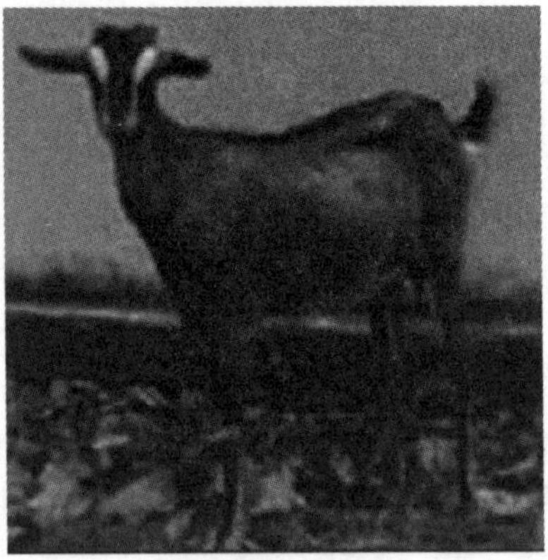

Raighari doe

II. Body measurements (adult goats)

Raighari goats are medium in size and is usually smaller than Ganjam goats and bigger as well as heavier than Black Bengal goats(Kornel *et al.,* 2006).

Traits (cm)	Male	Female
Body length (L1)	48.7	33.5
Body length (L2)	58.9	42.5
Height at withers	65.6	59.0
Chest girth or circumference	70.3	63.0

Paunch girth or abdomen girth	85.3	79.0
Neck girth	39.3	41.5
Thigh girth	29.4	24.0
Head length	17.9	14.5
Horn length (Range: 5-17 cm)	11.2	8.5
Ear length (Range: 12-15 cm)	13.6	12.0
Tail length	12.0	11.5

(L1: point of wither to hip joint; L2: hip joint to shoulder joint)

III. Body weights

Average body weight	Male	Female
Adult weight (kg)	27.0	25.5

IV. Reproductive and productive characteristics: The average age at sexual maturity and first kidding are 10-12 months and 15-18 months, respectively. Most of the reproductive and productive characteristics of this breed are similar to Narayanpatna goats.

(Kornel *et al.*, 2006)

13. GHUMUSARI GOATS

Place of origin: Odisha

These types of goats are distributed in the western part of Ganjam district i.e. Bhanjanagar and its adjoining areas of erstwhile Ghumusar tehsil of Odisha (Patro *et al.,* 2007). The flock size vary from 5-25. These goats are reared under pasture grazing available in the local tract. Verma *et al.* (2015) reported that these goats are also available in villages of Khandamal disitrict of Odisha. Animals are kept on pasture grazing.

I. Phenotypic characteristics

Color -Usually black, light brown to black brown with dark brown belly, medium in size.

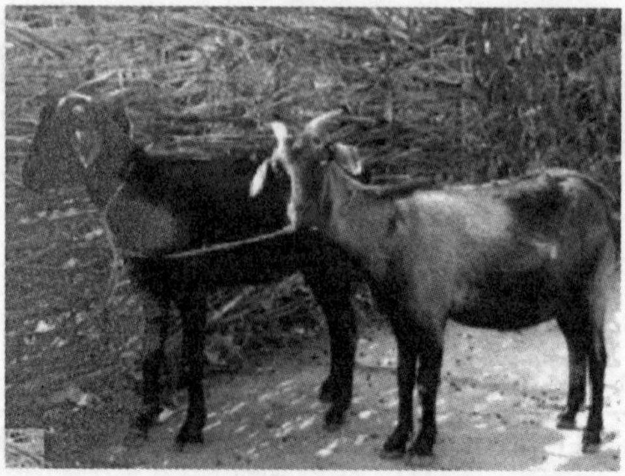

(Adopted from Verma *et al.*, 2015)

II. Body measurements (adult goats)

The Ghumusar goats grow faster than the Black Bengal type but the body weight is similar or a little less than Ganjam goats i.e. intermediate of body size between Black Bengal and Ganjam goats and is famous for excellent meat quality and early maturity however, it has birth weight higher Bengal type goats.

Traits (cm)	Male	Female
Body length	62.14	57.14
Height at withers	63.00	58.86
Chest girth or circumference	68.29	62.64
Paunch girth or Abdomen girth	71.00	66.46
Face length	14.86	13.95
Horn length	12.29	7.23
Ear length	14.14	13.28
Tail length	13.29	11.75

III. Body weights

Average body weight (kg)	Male	Female
3-6 months weight	8.60	8.15
7-12 months weight	13.25	12.07
Adult weight	20.86	19.88

(Verma *et al.*, 2011)

Patro *et al.* (2007) also reported that the body weight of these goats at birth, 3, 6, 9 and 12 month of age are 1.75, 7.14, 10.18, 13.01 and 17.05 kg, respectively.

IV. Reproductive and productive characteristics

These goats are as prolific as Black Bengal type goats but lower age at first kidding and kidding interval as compared to Ganjam goats. Does attain sexual maturity at about 12-18 months of age and natural mating is practiced in the flocks. The multiple births in terms of twins and triplets have been reported as 62.46 and 7.97%, respectively which are common from second kidding onwards.

(Verma *et al.*, 2011)

14. KALAHANDI GOATS

Home Tract: Odisha

These medium size goats are mainly found in Kalahandi and Nuapara district and adjoining areas of Odisha and are famous for their meat quality and adaptability under harsh climatic conditions like high temperature prevails in the native tract, which goes up to 48° C in summer. These goats are mostly reared by resource poor tribal community under range management system without any supplementation, housing and preventive health cover. The genetic biodiversity study of Verma *et al.* (2015) using Nei's DS genetic distance method indicated that Ghumusar and Kalahandi goats have highest genetic distance and plots separately from Ganjam and Black Bengal goats.

I. Phenotypic characteristics

Color - Mostly brown and white in colour and even mixed colors

Ear - Flat, leafy and drooping

Horns- Long, flat, upward and backward

Legs- Thin and cylindrical

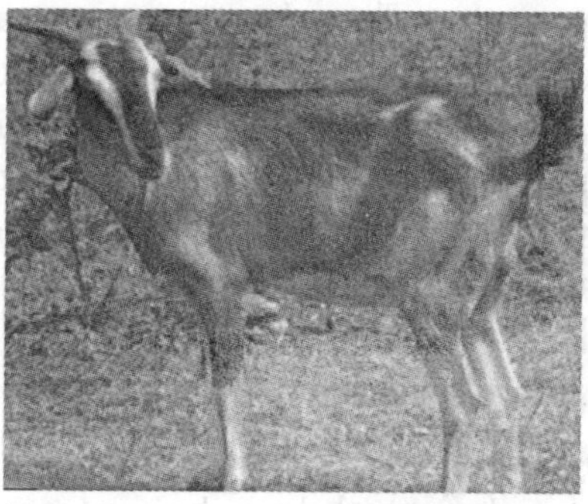

(Adopted from Verma *et al.*, 2015)

II. Body measurements (adult goats)

Traits (cm)	Male	Female
Body length	69.05	66.28
Height at withers	70.32	65.51
Chest girth or circumference	71.53	70.36
Paunch girth or Abdomen girth	73.84	74.87
Face length	17.89	15.29
Horn length	15.05	12.74
Ear length	15.74	15.01
Tail length	15.32	13.97

III. Reproductive and productive characteristics

The body weight at birth, 6 and 12 months age were reported to be 1.34, 7.84 and 15.23 kg, respectively. The reproduction potential of this goat is at par with Bengal type goats and higher incidence of multiple births viz. 26.54, 65.48 and 6.19% cases of single, twins and triplets were recorded in its native tract (Verma *et al.*, 2010, Mohanty *et al.*, 2011). In another study, Verma *et al.* (2015) reported that the body weights of adult male and females were 33.42 and 30.88 kg, 5.3% twins and 4.4% triplets and quadruplets. These goats are poor milkers.

15. KATHEWADI GOATS

Home Tract: Maharashtra

Mane *et al.* (2015) reported that the migratory nomadic shepherds from Kathewad region of Gujarat used to migrate to Dhulia district of Maharastra for grazing their animals being it an assured rain fall area with some goats as a leader. They donate some males while returning to their native place which were used as a buck for breeding of local does. This practice was followed for a long time, resulted into development of a new phenotypically stabilized breed, locally called Kathewadi goat breed. These goats thrive well by grazing on agricultural residues after harvesting season.

I. Phenotypic Characteristics

Color – Predominantly black coat, white spot on body and some brownish black colour with long hair, strong compact body

Forehaed- Convex type (93.33%) followed by straight and flat head (6.67%)

Ears- Long and pendulous

Horns- Present in 94.55% goats, remaining polled; twisted and long, spiral and curved (100%) shapes, oriented upward and backward (86.38%) and downward (13.62%)

Wattle - Present in males only (98.70%)

Beard- Present in males and females (9.30%)

Muzzle, Eye lids, Hooves- Black in color

Tail- Medium in length, tail types were slender (86.33%) and bunchy (13.67%), tail shapes were straight (98.33%) and curved (1.67%)

Udder and Teats- Well developed bowl shape udder with cylindrical teats having pointed tip

(Mane *et al.*, 2015)

II. Body measurements (adult goats)

Traits (cm)	Pooled irrespective of sex
Body length	73-75
Height at withers	80-85
Chest girth	75-80
Horn length	19.42 (15-17)
Ear length	23.18 (24-26)
Tail length	19.18 (16-19)
Teat length	12-14

III. Body weights

Average body weight (kg)	Pooled irrespective of sex
Birth weight	2.91
3m wt	11.45
6m wt	17.12
9m wt	21.51
12m wt	26.21

(Mane *et al.*, 2015)

IV. Reproductive and productive characteristics

The milk yield in this goat is observed to be 2-3 litres/day. The incidence of twins and triplets is about 45%, even though single kid is common in first kidding (Mane et al., 2015).

16. KAROLI GOATS

The breed derives its name from its native habitat of 'Karoli' area of Rajasthan. The animals are also found in some parts of Gujarat. Karoli goats are compact medium-sized animals.

I. Phenotypic Characteristics

Color: Predominantly black coat color. However, few white, brown and spotted animals are also found

Horn: Both sexes have typical small cork screw horns pointed upward and backward

Ear: Long, broad, medium sized, leaf like drooping ears

Nose: Slightly Roman

Hair: Body is covered fairly and densely with short and coarse hair

Udder and Teats: Moderately developed udder with conical shaped teats

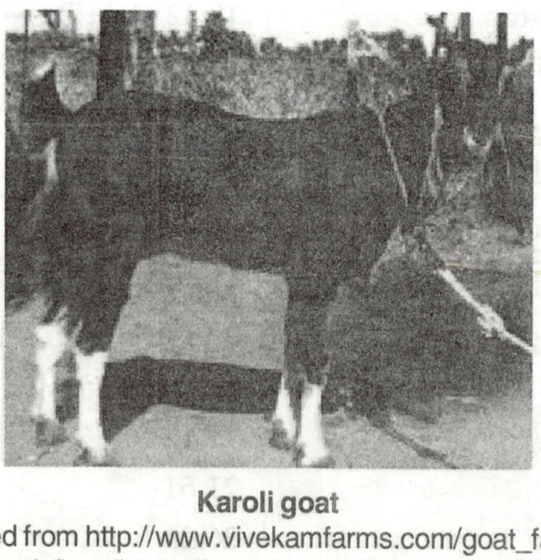

Karoli goat

(Adopted from http://www.vivekamfarms.com/goat_farming/goat_breeds/karoli; http://www.al-nwader.com/vb/t6342.html)

II. Body Measurements (adult goats)

Traits (cm)	Male	Female
Body length	65	66
Chest girth	70.5	71.5

III. Body weights (kg)

Average body weight	Male	Female
Adult weight (kg)	30	32
Birth weight is about 2.0 kg		

IV. Reproductive and productive characteristics

The age at first kidding is 19-20 months and the litter size is one kid per birth. The breed is well suited to stall feeding. Average yield varies around 1.5 kg and the lactation length is about 110 days (http://www.vivekamfarms.com/goat_farming/goat_breeds/karoli; http://www.al-nwader.com/vb/t6342.html).

17. SOJAT

Home Tract : Rajasthan

Sojat goats originate from Rajasthan in India. Mostly present in between the belt of Sojat, Aau (Phalodi), Pipar, Jodhpur and other small part of Rajasthan. It is crossbred of Jamunapari goat of Uttar Pradesh, therefore the animals of this breed looks like a Jamunapari goats. The breed is famous for white color and good height and health. Sojat goats are good for meat purpose and are primarily farmed for its meat as the milk yield is low. The milk production is about 65 kg per lactation period. The breed is suitable for stall feed goat farming.

I. Phenotypic characteristics

Color - Great variation in coat color but they are generally white in color with pink skin. Occasionally patches of tan or black are found on the body

Ear - Ears are very long, flat and drooping

Horn - Mostly absent in both sexes.

Tail - Short and thin tail

Hair - Thin growth of hair is present on the body

Udder and Teats - Well developed round shaped udder with large conical teats

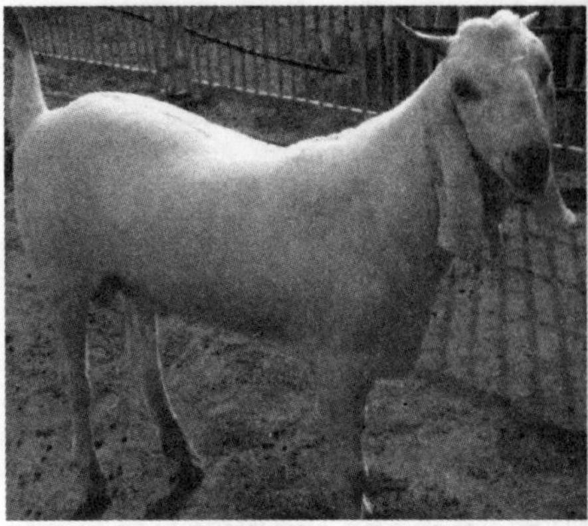
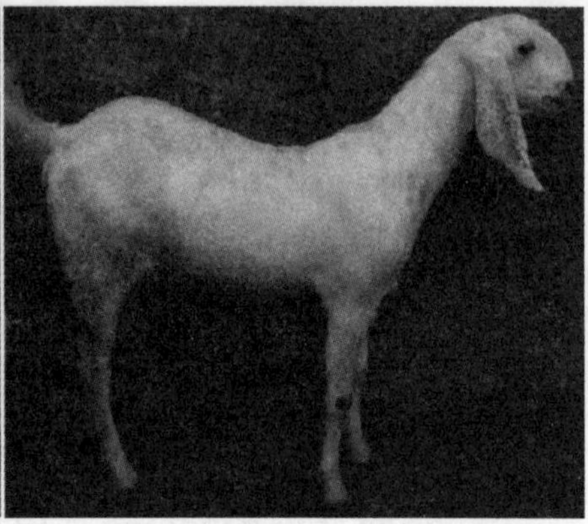

Sojat buck **Sojat doe**

Courtsey: Naeem qureshi goat supplier, Farah, Mathura

II. Body measurements (adult goats)

Traits (cm)	Male	Female
Body Length (cm)	80	78
Chest Girth (cm)	85	80

III. Body weights

Body weight	Male	Female
Adult weight (kg)	50-60	40-50

IV. Reproductive and productive characteristics

The milk yield is relatively small, about 0.5 kg per day, with an average milk yield of 65 kg over a 120 day lactation period (http://sojatgoatsindia.blogspot.ae/2011/03/sojat-goats-in-india.html). However, higher production of average daily yield varies from 1.0 to 1.5 kg per day with a total lactation yield of about 175 kg is also reported (http://goatindia.com/category-sojat.html). Usually doe kids twice in 12 to 14 months, giving birth to single in 40% while twins in 60% cases (http://sojatgoatsindia.blogspot.ae /2011/03/sojat-goats-in-india.html).

18. BATTISI

Home Tract: Rajasthan, Uttar Pradesh

The Battisi breed of goat is originated during due course of time by cross breeding of three recognized goat breeds i.e. Jamunapari, Sirohi and Jakhrana. The animals of this breed possess the characteristic features of three goat breeds viz., body confirmation like Sirohi, milk production potential like Jamunapari and Jakhrana goats (Singh *et al.*, 2014). The animals of this breed have a potential to perform better in spite of adverse climatic variables. Thus due to its better production potential, the animals of this breed fetch better price as compared to the animals of other breed in their home tract.

I. **Phenotypic characteristics**

Color: Mostly white coat color with black and brown patches on face, chest, shoulder, abdomen and legs. Few animals are of mixed color

Nose: Roman type

Ears: Medium size (15-20 cm) drooping ears

Udder and Teats: Large sized udder with conical teats

Hair: Small hairs throughout the body however, log hairs on neck, back and legs

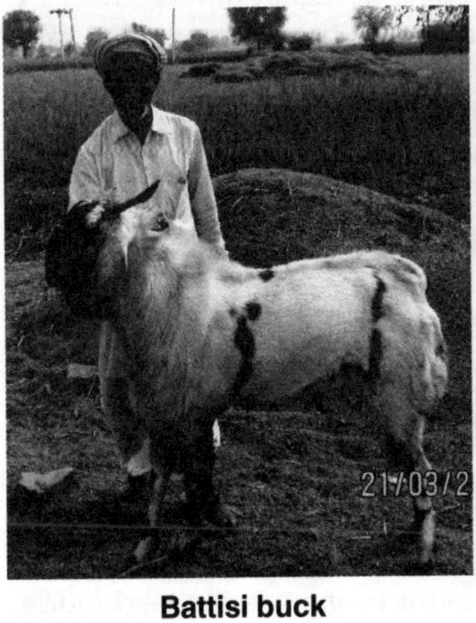

Battisi buck

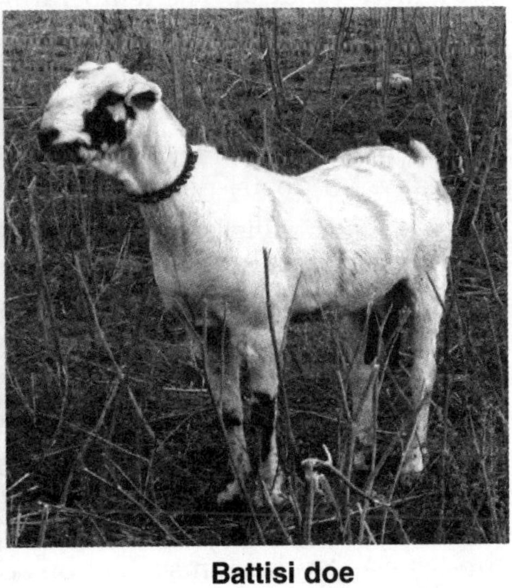

Battisi doe

Courtesy: Singh *et al.* (2014)

II. Body weights

Average body weight (kg)	Male	Female
6 m body weight	16.0	13.0
12 m body weight (kg)	30.0	25.0
Adult (2 yrs) body weight	50.0	38.0

III. Reproductive and productive characteristics

Trait	Characteristics
Age of first kidding (months)	18-20
Kidding interval (months)	About 12
Twining rate (%)	50
Average daily milk production (liter)	1.5
Lactation length (days)	200

(Singh *et al.*, 2014)

19. BUNDELKHANDI GOATS

Home Tract: Uttar Pradesh / Madhya Pradesh

Bundelkhandi goats are mainly distributed in Bundelkhand region which encompasses the Chitrakut, Banda, Jhansi, Jalaun, Hamirpur, Mahoba and Lalitpur districts of Uttar Pradesh and Chhatarpur, Tikamgarh, Damoh, Sagar Datia, Satna, Panna and Gawalior districts of Madhya Pradesh. The temperature of this region ranged from 1°C in winter to more than 40°C in summer and the occurrence of rains and drought is highly irregular. However, the purest form of Bundelkhandi goats is found in Datia district of Madhya Pradesh and Jhanshi district of Uttar Pradesh. Landless and marginal farmers rear generally 1-5 goats, people of Pal community rear 20-40 goats and sheep in many villages of this region. Along with this type of goats, the different grades of Jakhrana, Jamunapari, Sirohi and barbari breeds are reared by farmers in this region. The Indigenous goats are predominantly reared by extensive farmers and mixed crosses among small holders. In general, farmers favour the crossbreeding for upgrading of local goats (Bhusan *et al.*, 2010; Verma *et al.*, 2010; Annual report, NBAGR: 2010-11). The productivity of these goats is reported to be much lower than their actual production potential (Mishra *et al.*, 2012, Singh *et al.*, 2014) that is mainly attributed to subsistence production system on account of inadequate feed-fodder and breeding practices.

I. Phenotypic characteristics

The Bundelkhandi goats are able to survive in very low and high temperature in different seasons of Bundelkhand region due to its black color and long legs. Long and sturdy legs also make them suitable for long walk in the rocky terrain of this region.

Color - Jet black coat color

Eyelids and Muzzle - Black color

Legs - Long

Face- Narrow

Nose- Roman type

Hairs- Long hairs on the whole body

Ears – Long, curly, pendulous

Tail – Bushy

(Bhusan *et al.*, 2010; Verma *et al.*, 2010)

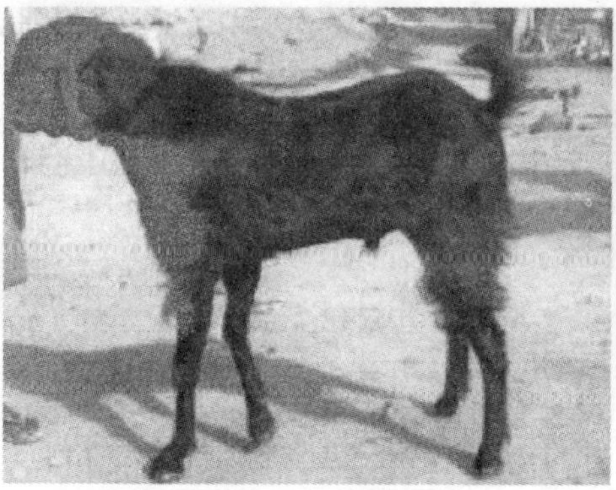

Bundelkhandi buck

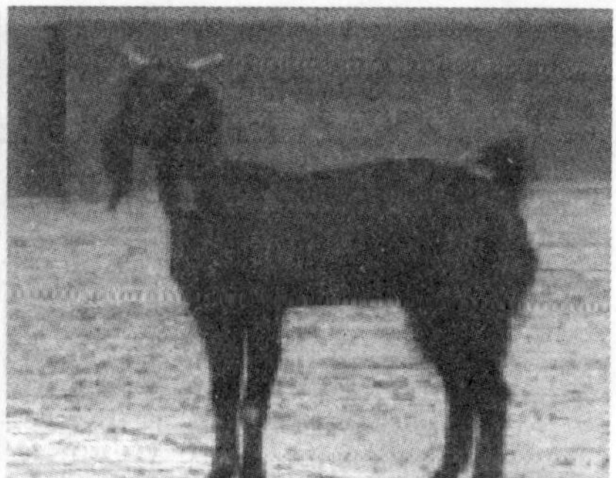

Bundelkhandi doe

(Adopted from Annual report, NBAGR, 2010-11)

II. Body measurements

These goats are large sized, hardy, tall and compact body and sustain extreme climatic conditions of its habitat and rough terrain. The measurements of farm reared goats are higher than goats reared under field management conditions.

Traits (cm)	Farm bred		Grazing/field		Overall	
	Male	Female	Male	Female	Male	Female
Body length	80.00	72.61	78.10	71.93	78.42	72.24
Height at withers	78.50	73.17	77.00	71.63	77.25	72.34
Chest/Heart girth	75.50	72.43	77.40	72.11	77.08	72.26
Paunch girth	68.50	72.52	79.50	72.26	77.67	72.38
Face length	19.00	16.96	18.40	12.88	18.50	14.80
Horn length	14.50	9.63	14.80	12.67	14.75	11.53
Ear length	18.50	18.78	19.20	19.33	19.08	19.08
Tail length	16.00	15.52	17.20	15.67	17.00	15.60

III. Body weights

Management conditions and sex	Farm bred		Grazing/field		Overall	
	Male	Female	Male	Female	Male	Female
Average Adult weight (kg)	37.50	33.13	39.70	32.90	39.33	33.01

(Bhusan *et al.*, 2010; Verma *et al.*, 2010; Annual report, NBAGR, 2010-11)

IV. Reproductive and productive characteristics

These goats are good for meat and milk. Under good feeding and management conditions, the peak milk yield of many goats reaches up to 2.8 lit/day with 220 days lactation length. The recorded milk yield at 90 and 120 days are 53.57 and 76.72 litres, respectively (Verma *et al.*, 2010).

20. JAUNPURI/ JAFRABADI GOATS

Home Tract: Uttar Pradesh

The Jaunpuri/Jafrabadi goats is dual purpose goats mainly distributed in Sultanpur, Jaunpur and Faizabad districts of eastern Uttar Pradesh and is dual-purpose goats reared for milk and meat (Singh *et al.*, 2010a, 2010b; Verma *et al*, 2010). These goats have been probably developed by crossing Jamunapari male with nondescript females of this region before independence but remain neglected from the attention of scientific communities. However, as a result of close breeding the germplasm of this breed has been persisted and established well. The goats are usually reared by small, marginal and landless farmers under extensive system/grazing on natural shrubs and herbs and mainly housed in thatch structures. The goat farmers in the native tract were generally selling the goats through commission agents to the wholesalers and meat dealers in the local market. The marketing cost per goat comes around Rs. 69.28 in small (1-5 goats) followed by Rs. 66.57 in medium (6-10 goats) and Rs. 64.52 in large (more than 10 goats) flocks. The farmers usually gets 70.25% share for their produce whereas middlemen/agents, wholesalers and meat dealers receives 12, 8.25 and 9.50% share, respectively (Srivastava and Saraswat, 2006).

I. Body measurements (adult goats)

The goats of Jaunpuri breed are smaller to Jamunapari but larger to Barbari goat in size.

Traits (cm)	Male	Female
Body length	56.50	50.27
Height at withers	70.67	63.26
Chest girth or circumference	71.50	66.20

II. Body weights

Average body weight (kg)	Male	Female
Adult weight	34.83	24.47

III. Reproductive and productive characteristics

Goats are bred through natural service and twinning is very common.

Traits	Average age/ Remarks
Age at first heat/estrous (months)	12.423
Age at first kidding (months)	18.21
Service period (days)	55.63
Kidding interval (days)	205.36
Gestation length (days)	149.72
Litter size (%)	
Twins	61.0-77.0

Milk Yield	In Jaunpur district, goats are milked for about 4-5 months after kidding with an average of 1.0-1.5 lit milk/day, whereas in Faizabad district, the goats yield only 0.5-0.7 lit milk/day and are milked for 2.5-3.0 months only.

(Singh *et al.*, 2010 a, b; Verma *et al.*, 2010)

21. BAREILLY GOATS

Verma *et al.* (2010) opined that these goats are found in Rohilkhand area Bareilly district of Uttar Pradesh and are reared mainly for meat purpose. The twinning rates in these goats have been observed as high as more than 50%.

I. Phenotypic characteristics

Color - Black coat with hair tuft in breech

Nose- Roman type

Ears- Broad and pendulous

Horns - Twisted and short

II. Body weights

Average body weight (kg)	Pooled irrespective of sex
Birth weight	2-3
At weaning	8-10
6-9 months weight	10-15
12 months weight	20-25
Adult (more than 12 months) weight	35-40

(Das, 2008; Verma *et al.*, 2010)

22. CHAUGARKHA GOATS or HILL GOATS

Home Tract: Uttarakhand

The name Chaugarkha has been derived from the name of the area Chaugarkha Patti *i.e.* Chitai to Dania in Almora district from where this breed has originated. The breed is distributed in Almora district and adjoining area of Bageshwar, Pithoragarh and Nainital district of Uttarakhand (Singh and Barwal, 2007, 2009; Singh *et al.*, 2010; Verma *et al.*, 2010). Chaugarkha is a new strain evolved in the Kumaon region due to repeated cross breeding between different breeds of goats. It sustain well in its home tract due to its hardiness on the denuded cliffs where other agricultural activities are barely profitable. Joshi (1992) reported that Chaugarkha goats thrives well in most densely inhabited areas with maximum agronomic pressure at 3000-5000 m altitude, when other exotic plain goat breeds are unable to adopt. This goat is hardy, disease resistant, small sized and flourishes in its home tract with steep escarpments.

Farmers rear this goat along with some other non-descript goats with a herd size of 8-12 goats. However, medium sized herd have 20-30 goats. The goats are reared in an unorganized, semi-feral system of husbandry. The kids are reared with their mothers and suckle them during early life and are also fed grasses and tree leaves up to three month of age, and thereafter they are allowed to browse along with the herd. The goats in smaller flocks are mostly housed along with bovines while the flocks having more than 5 goats are housed separately in closed type poorly ventilated pens. The goats are either marketed as live-animals or slaughtered at maturity for own consumption and for sacrificial purposes in religious rituals. Marketing of live animals is unorganized and trading or prices are decided on live body weight basis (Singh and Barwal, 2007, 2009).

I. Phenotypic characteristics

The Chaugarkha is a small size meat goat breed, reared mainly for meat purpose.

Color - The coat colour of this breed varies from black, fawn and white. Hooves and dew claws are grey in color; horns are ash grey to grey in color

Head - Convex, small in length

Forehead - Small to medium

Ear – Medium and horizontal

Horn - Straight outwards

Muzzle –Tapering in nature

Eyes- Alert

Nose- Roman

Top line- Almost straight

Flank- Moderate in size and not too wide

Thigh- Lean and not well developed

Legs – Small, lean and straight legs squarely set under body

Tail- Thin, short in length and curled wrapped

Udder- Small with well-set small pointed teats

(Singh and Barwal, 2007, 2009)

II. Body measurements (adult goats)

Devendra and Burns (1983) reported that based on height and withers, goats can be classified as large (more than 65 cm), small (51-65 cm) and dwarf (less than 50 cm). Thus the Chaugarkha goat can be grouped under small breed and are having a lean body and reared for meat purpose (Singh and Barwal, 2007, 2009).

Traits (cm)	Male	Female
Body length	54.67	54.71
Height at withers	54.60	53.97
Chest girth	59.57	60.76
Paunch girth	63.33	66.82
Face length	14.53	14.56
Horn length	8.97	6.80
Ear length	13.55	13.73
Tail length	11.88	11.34

III. Body weights

Average body weight (kg)	Male	Female
0-3 m weight	6.20 (pooled)	
4-9 m weight	8.03 (pooled)	
7-9 m weight	12.37	10.52
10-12 m weight	12.88	11.12
Adult weight	18.18	17.61

IV. Reproductive and productive characteristics

The Chaugarkha goat seems to have good reproduction potential in terms of early sexual maturity. The breeding bucks are maintained at all times in the flocks resulting in early mating of most of the females. Majority of the flocks of larger size maintain males for breeding and of smaller size got mated the does with breeding bucks from other flocks. Only a few male kids were selected for breeding purposes and others are disposed off or slaughtered for meat purpose at an early age and almost all the females are retained. Only old does are sold for meat purpose.

Traits	Average age / Remarks
Age at sexual maturity (months)	10-12
Age at first kidding (months)	16-18
Kidding interval (months)	kid once a year
Twinning	Frequently occurs in healthy goats
Average daily milk yield	Does do not yield any appreciable quantity of milk except for nourishing the kids.
Meat	Meat is course and devoid of fat. Breed is widely used for sacrificial purpose.

(Singh and Barwal, 2007, 2009; Singh *et al.*, 2010, Verma *et al.*, 2010)

23. UDAIPURI GOATS

Home Tract: Uttarakhand

The Udaipuri goats are found in Ajmer and Udaipur patties in the Western Himalayan region of Uttarakhand and reared for meat production. These patties have been named on the basis of peoples migrated from Ajmer and Udaipur districts of Rajasthan to the above mentioned areas before centuries. Hence the name 'Udaipuri' has been derived and the main distribution areas are Dugadda, Pokhal, Kandi, Yamkeshwar, Devrana and adjoining areas of Pauri Garhwal Districts (Singh and Barwal, 2009; Barwal *et al.*, 2010 a, b; Verma *et al.*, 2010). The climate is generally semi temperate to temperate. The average flock size in their home tract is ranging from 10-50 goats. Udaipuri goats are managed under unorganized semi feral systems of management. Farmers hardly fed any concentrates to the goats. Kids are also allowed for browsing along with their mothers after 3 months of age. The kids and adult goats of more than 5 per flock are housed together after browsing hours during night in closed pens without ventilation. The goats in smaller flocks are housed along with bovines. Due to the cold weather conditions of the native tract, stored leaves collected from forests are used as bedding materials and are replaced at 2-3 days intervals for winter protection of goats (Barwal *et al.*, 2010 a, b).

I. Phenotypic characteristics

Color - Coat color is tan, body is covered with short hairs, which are not shorn. Horn color is ash grey to grey, hooves and dew claws are grey in color

Head - Convex, small in length

Forehead - Small to medium

Ear – Medium and pendulous

Horn – Curved and backward down

Muzzle – Tapering in nature

Nose- Roman

Eyes- Alert

Top line- Almost straight

Flank- Moderate in size and not too wide

Legs – Small, lean and straight legs squarely set under the body

Thigh- Lean and well developed

Tail- Thin, short in length and wrapped

Udder- Small size with well-set small pointed teats

(Barwal *et al.*, 2010 a, b)

II. Body measurements (adult goats)

These goats are small in size with compact body.

Traits (cm)	Male	Female
Body length	61.21	60.82
Height at withers	62.03	59.10
Chest girth	71.57	70.96
Forehead length	15.97	15.09
Horn length	16.05	12.17
Ear length	14.73	14.44
Tail length	12.76	11.87

III. Body weights

Average body weight	Male	Female
Adult weight (kg)	24.67	22.10

(Barwal *et al.*, 2010 a,b)

IV. Reproductive and productive characteristics

The breeding bucks are maintained at all times in the flocks and the farmers exercise no control over mating. Majority of the flocks of larger size maintain males for breeding. Only a few male kids were selected for breeding purposes and others are disposed off or slaughtered for meat purpose at an early age and almost all the females are retained. Only old does are sold for meat purpose. Udaipuri goats seem to have good reproduction potential.

Traits	Remarks
Age at sexual maturity	10-12 months
Kidding interval	Kidding once a year
Twinning	Fairly frequent in healthy goats
Average daily milk yield	Does do not yield any appreciable quantity of milk except for nourishing the kids
Meat	Meat is coarse and devoid of fat. Breed is widely used for sacrificial purpose

(Singh and Barwal, 2009; Barwal *et al.*, 2010 a, b; Verma *et al.*, 2010)

24. TARAI GOATS

Home Tract: Uttrakhand

These goats are seen in rural households of Tarai region of the Uttarakhand state and are reared for milk and meat (Verma *et al.*, 2010). It thrives well due to its hardiness in high rainfall and hot humid climate of the area. The color pattern ranges from black, tan, fawn, white and spots of these colors to others. These goats are small to medium in size yielding 1-1.5 kg milk/day from well set udder with small teats. These goats kid once a year with 2-3 kids reflecting the good potential for multiple births (Verma *et al.*, 2010).

25. ASSAM HILL GOATS

Home Tract: Assam

This goat is widely distributed in Assam and other hilly areas of adjacent North Eastern states. This goat is famous for meat production and is a poor milk yielder. Selected animals of this breed maybe suggested for utilization by the poor farmers of Assam and its adjoining areas for their economic upliftment. These goats are usually maintained by marginal farmers and they act as a source of insurance in the time of need (Zeshmarani *et al.*, 2007; Annual report, ICAR Research complex for NEH, 2008-09, 2009-10 and 2010-11).

I. Phenotypic characteristics

Small in size and well-proportioned body

Color - Predominant colors are black, black and white, and brown with patches of different colors in the body

Ears- Three types of ears are observed with horizontal medium-sized type is dominant followed by erect and pendulous

Horns- Thick and small sized (7.7 cm), black, directed upward and backward in females and straight upward in males

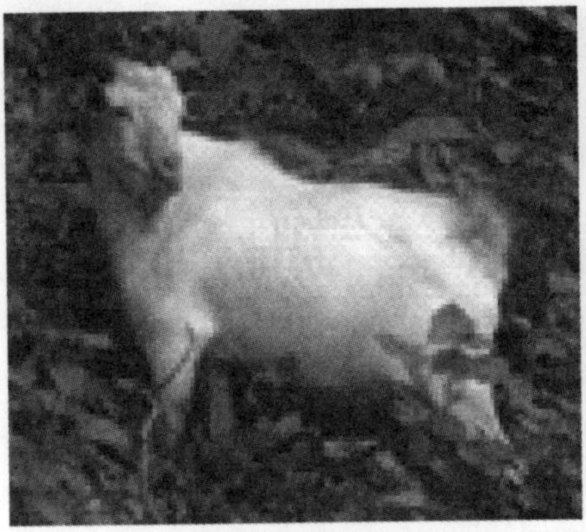
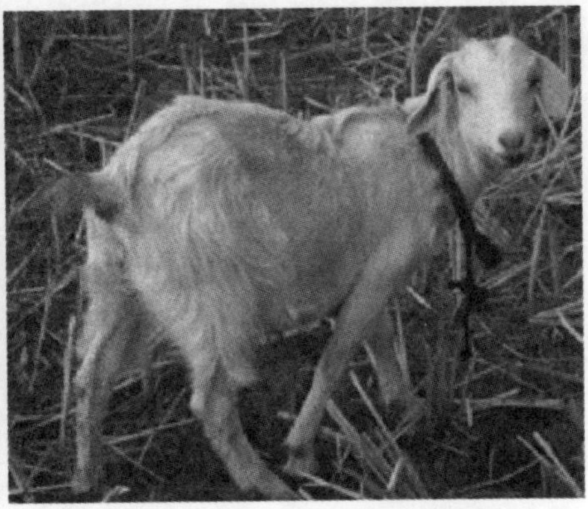

Assam Hill Goat - Male   Assam Hill Goat - Female
(Courtesy: Dr. Pranjal Borah, Assam)

II. Body measurements (adult goats)

Traits (cm)	Pooled (irrespective of sex)
Body length	84.23
Height at withers	55.50
Heart girth	63.85
Abdominal girth	77.80
Paunch girth	69.26
Head length	17.50
Neck length	36.50
Horn length	7.70
Ear length	12.59
Tail length	10.25

III. Body weights

Average body weight (kg)	Male	Female	Overall
Birth weight (Type of birth- Single)	1.71	1.52	-
Birth weight (Type of birth- Twins)	1.49	1.35	-

Birth weight (Type of birth- Triplet)	1.30	1.19	-
Birth weight (Overall)	1.58	1.39	1.48
3 m weight	6.87	6.1	6.48
6 m weight	10.26	8.93	9.32
9 m weight	11.73	9.45	10.41
12 m weight	14.20	11.91	12.93
Adult weight	-	-	21.18

III. Reproductive and productive characteristics

This goat is famous for meat production. The marketable age varies from 7 to 11 months and weight varies from 8-12 kg.

Traits	Average age (days)
Age at puberty	260-270
Age at first conception	279-295
Age at first kidding	437-447
Kidding interval	257.2
Gestation period	147
Prolificacy (%)	
Single	58.56
Twins	38.45
Triplets	2.98
Milk production (kg)	Negligible

(Zeshmarani *et al.*, 2007; Annual report, ICAR Research complex for NEH, 2008-09, 2009-10, 2010-11)

26. NON-PASHMINA GOATS

Home Tract: Jammu and Kashmir

This type of goats is mainly found in Leh, Khaltsey and Nubra blocks of Ladakh and are commonly reared for meat, manure, wool and milk.

I. Phenotypic characteristics

Color - Coat color is predominantly white

Horns- Long, curved, pointed backward and outward

Hairs- Long hairs on the whole body

Ears- Medium in length

Tail - Bushy

II. Body measurements (adult goats)

This goat is smaller in size.

Traits (inches)	Pooled (irrespective of sex)
Body length	25.02
Height at withers	21.98
Heart girth or circumference	28.05
Trunk girth	34.11
Horn length	11.23
Ear length	4.75
Tail length	4.36

III. Body weights

Average body weight	Pooled (irrespective of sex)
Adult weight (kg)	26.78

IV. Reproductive and productive characteristics

Traits	Remarks
Age at first kidding (days)	785
Kidding interval (days)	350
Prolificacy (%)	5-10
Milk Yield (lit/day)	0.1 to 0.25

(Roy *et al.*, 2007; Verma *et al.*, 2010)

27. TERESSA GOATS

Home Tract: Andaman and Nicobar Islands

Teressa goats are an indigenous species of Andaman and Nicobar Islands and are reared mainly for meat purpose. The name "Teressa" have been coined from the Island Teressa, a unique Island among Nicobar group of Islands. Teressa goats are mainly distributed in tribes of Teressa, Katchal and Champin Islands which is Nicobar group of Islands (Jeyakumar *et al.*, 2000; Yadav *et al.*, 2000; Anthra, 2006; Verma *et al.*, 2010). For these three islands, the herd composition revealed that the average holding of goats per family was found to be 11.67, 3.0, 3.60, respectively. Teressa goats were usually maintained under free range management system and can survive in hot and humid climate. Teressa goat is generally reared by the tribal farmers of Nicobar group of islands and it is an integral part of their tradition and culture. Sadana and Kaur (2011) reported that Teressa island has goats with high tolerance to saline water and are often termed as 'Teressa Goats' as a new strain. Anthra (2006) reported that the approximate population of these goats is about 2000-3000 in the tract. The population of goat in the Nicobar district in 2010 was only 8357 (Kundu *et al.*, 2010).

I. Phenotypic Characteristics:

Color - Brownish or dark tan or black or white in colour with white and black patches. Dorsal midline was lined by black hairs up to the tail. The presence of a white patch or line starting from inner canthus of both eyes or from eye brows and extending up to nostrils or mouth is the most prominent feature (Kundu *et al.*, 2010, Kundu *et al.*, 2014)

Muzzle, Eyelids and Hooves - Black color

Ear - Little erect and directed downwards

Horn - Large, flat at base and directed backwards

Beard and Wattle - Some goats, it is absent

Tail - Generally medium to long

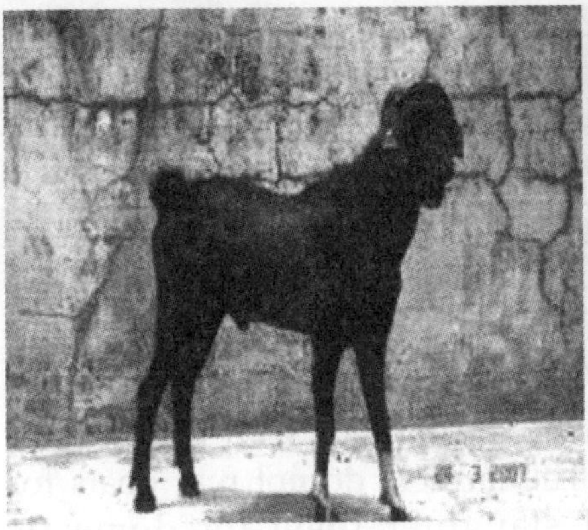

Teressa buck

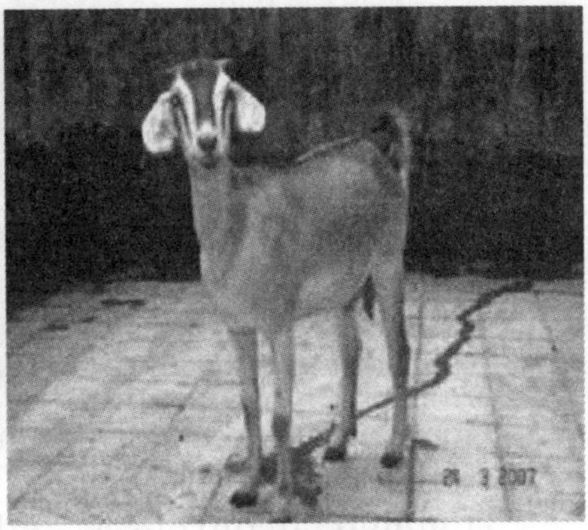

Teressa doe

(Adopted from http://cari.res.in/animal-ach/teressa%20goat.htm)

II. Body measurements

Majority of the goats appeared very tall compared to other local breeds, sturdy, healthy and timid in nature. The height of goats ranged from 26 to 32 inches and the castrated male reached even more than this height.

Traits (inches)	Male	Female
Body length	27.61	24.40
Height at withers	25.50	25.13
Chest girth	27.38	27.99
Paunch/abdomen girth	31.22	32.14
Neck girth	14.20	11.84
Head length	7.20	6.14
Ear length	4.81	5.20
Ear width	2.37	2.60
Ear girth	4.69	4.96
Horn length	5.64	4.06
Leg length	20.30	18.99
Tail length	4.62	5.05
Hoof girth	6.60	5.99

III. Body weights

Average body weight	Male	Female
Adult weight (kg)	34.92	32.36

(Jeyakumar *et al.*, 2000; Yadav *et al.*, 2000; Anthra, 2006; Verma *et al.*, 2010)

IV. Reproductive and productive characteristics

Goats are reared mainly for meat consumption with some farmer rears for milk consumption. The farmers do not rear goats for commercial purposes and slaughter them for domestic consumption during different festivals, sports or community functions. Drum like musical instrument is also being prepared by using skin of this goat. Normally goats are slaughtered at 14.1 months with an average live weight at slaughter of 45.7 kg. They generally give birth to twins and triplets. These goats are resistant to common diseases (Jeyakumar *et al.*, 2000; Yadav *et al.*, 2000).

28. LOCAL ANDAMAN GOATS

Home Tract: Andaman and Nicobar Islands

Local Andaman goats were usually maintained under semi intensive system management system and goat farming serves as an asset for landless, marginal farmers and tribal of Andaman & Nicobar Islands (Yadav *et al.*, 2000; Anthra, 2006; Verma *et al.*, 2010).

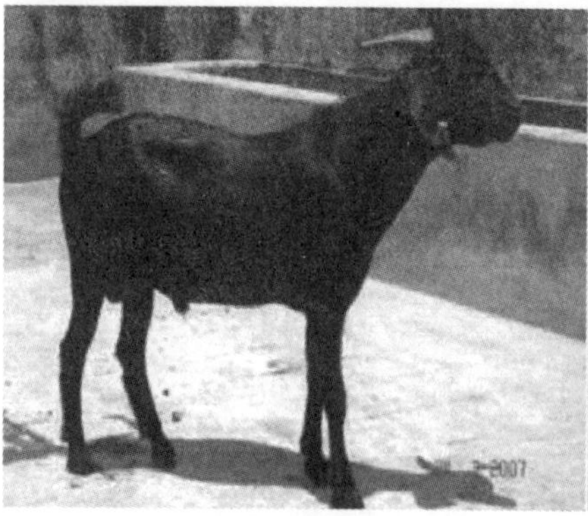

Local Andaman buck

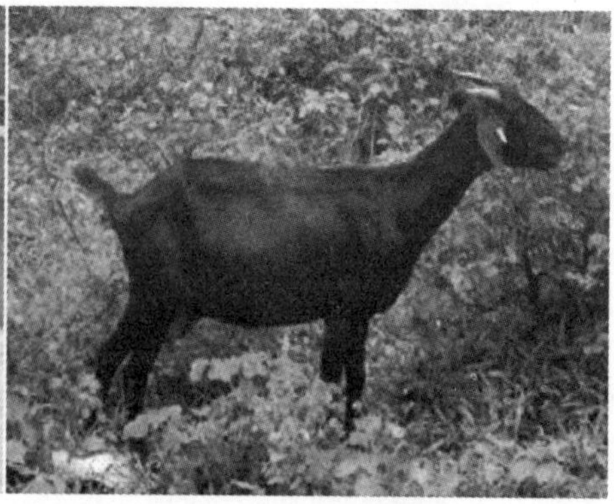

Local Andaman doe

I Body measurements

Traits (inches)	Male	Female
Body length	21.76	21.28
Height at withers	22.59	22.28
Chest girth	25.98	24.09
Paunch/abdomen girth	26.63	30.06
Neck girth	13.07	11.31
Head length	6.80	6.59
Ear length	5.33	5.18
Ear width	3.00	3.04
Ear girth	4.95	4.79
Horn length	3.96	2.40
Leg length	18.38	18.24
Tail length	4.77	4.18
Hoof girth	5.98	5.68
Scrotal circumference	7.30	-
Udder circumference	-	8.73

II. Body weights

Average body weight	Male	Female
Adult weight (kg)	28.21	23.45

(Jeyakumar *et al.*, 2000; Yadav *et al.*, 2000)

29. SINGHAREY GOATS

Home Tract: Sikkim

Singharey goats are found throughout Sikkim especially more concentrated in western district and mainly reared for meat purposes. These goats since ancient times have been surviving in Himalayan terrain and rocky mountains of the state and provide livelihood security of small and marginal farmers even under odd climatic conditions. Goats are managed under mostly on semi-extensive system of rearing with grazing in hill forests from morning to evening and during night hours; they are kept in temporary shelters. Shelters are made of bamboo sticks and wooden logs with raised floor 3-4 feet from ground. Few goats are also reared under stall feeding conditions.

I Phenotypic characteristics

These goats are phenotypically distinct from the other populations of NEH region i.e. Bengal type, Assam local and longfiber goats.

Color - Brown, fawn and black and white; distinct feature is presence of white stripes on face that extends from base of the horns up to muzzle and upper jaw. Under belly is generally light brown or white, medially white or black in legs, black top line was found in many goats. Breeding buck has prominent black color ring around neck which is absent/poorly developed in castrated males.

Head - Medium in length

Ear – Short to medium, semi-pendulous with round tip and have black or white margin on the apical half. Rudimentary ears found in few cases.

Legs– Short, stout; hair seen in thigh region in few goats

Udder and Teats– Moderately developed with small conical shaped teats

(Verma *et al.*, 2015)

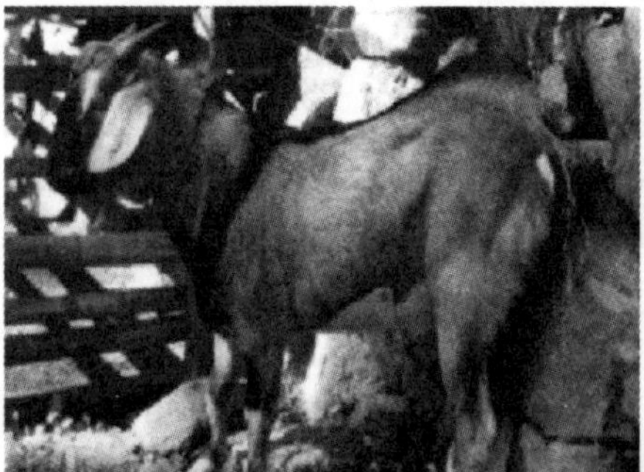

Singharey buck

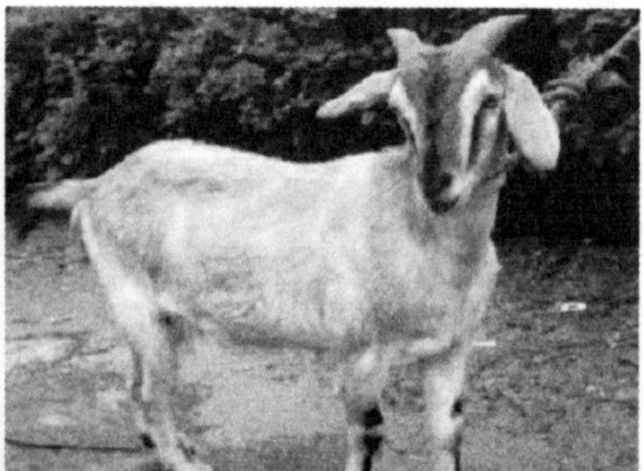

Singharey doe

II Body measurements

These goats forms the major part of Sikkim goat population

Traits (cm)	Male	Female
Body length	61.48	60.29
Height at withers	55.67	52.52
Chest girth	71.66	67.98
Paunch/abdomen girth	76.47	74.52
Face length	17.20	16.16
Ear length	12.92	13.48
Horn length	14.58	8.84
Tail length	11.89	10.88

III Body weight

Average body weight (kg)	Male	Female
Adultweight	27.33	31.03

(Verma *et al.*, 2015)

IV Reproductive and productive characteristics

The bucks reach maturity and ready to serve at 9-10 months age. Female kids attain maturity at around 9-12 months. Usually males castrated at 3 months of age for better growth. Breeding is done by natural mating and breeding bucks are genetically poor and are associated with reproductive problems. Twinning is very common in these goats. The milk yield is 300-500 ml/day, though milking is not practiced on regular basis and kids are allowed to suckle.

□□□

Chapter 5

LIST OF RECOGNISED AND LESSER KNOWN SHEEP GERMPLASM IN INDIA

List of recognized sheep breeds in India

S. No.	Name	Home Tract	Body size	Utility	Image
1.	Balangir	Odisha	Medium	Extremely coarse, hairy and open	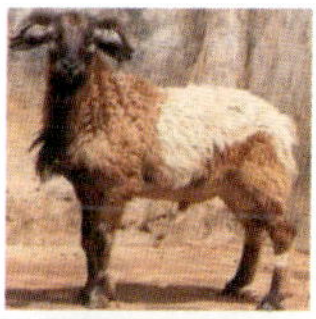
2.	Bellary	Karnataka	Medium	Extremely coarse, hairy and open	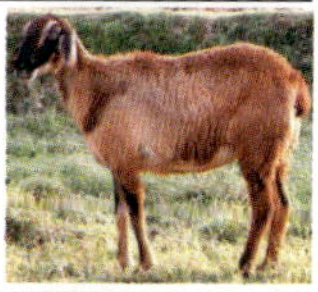
3.	Bhakarwal	Jammu and Kashmir	Medium	coarse and open	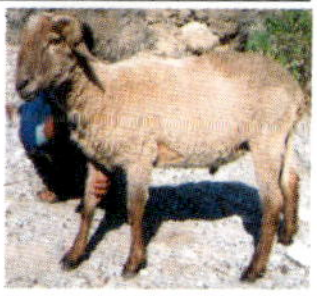
4.	Bonpala	Sikkim	Large	Coarse, hairy and open	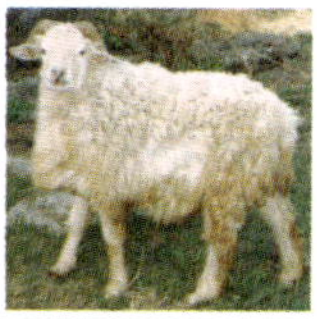
5.	Changthangi	Jammu and Kashmir	Large	Good carpet/ medium apparel quality	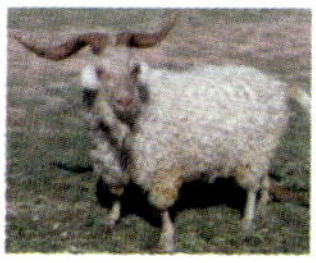

6.	Chokla (Chapper, Shekhawati)	Rajasthan	Medium	Finest carpet-wool type	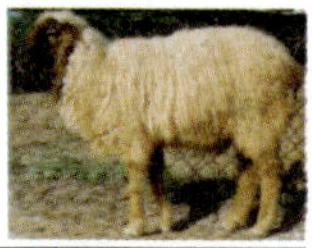
7.	Chottnagpuri	Jharkhand	Small	Coarse, hairy and open	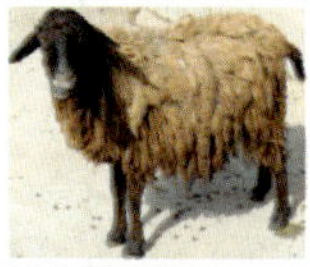
8.	Coimbatore (Kurumbai)	Tamil Nadu	Medium	Coarse, hairy and open	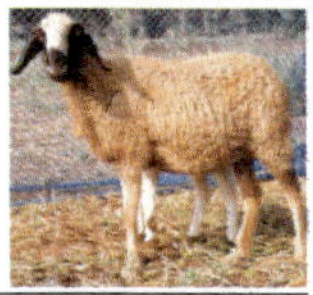
9.	Deccani	Andhra Pradesh and Maharashtra	Medium	Coarse, hairy and open	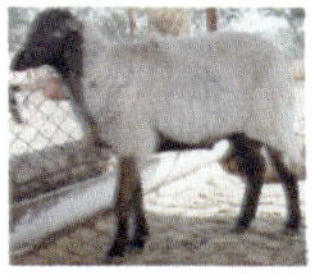
10.	Gaddi (Bhadarwah)	Himachal Pradesh	Medium	Relatively fine and dense	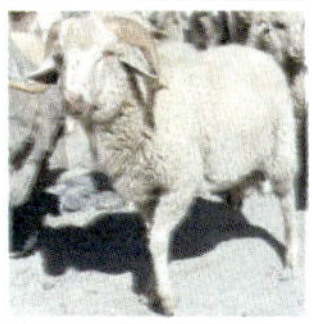
11.	Ganjam	Odisha	Medium	Hairy and short	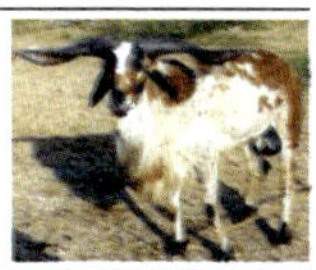
12.	Garole	West Bengal		Coarse and hairy (rough carpet quality)	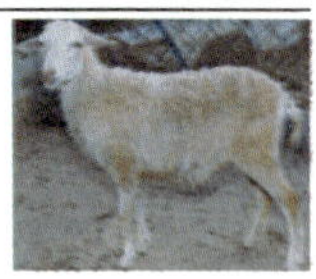
13.	Gurez	Jammu and Kashmir	Large (Largest sheep breed of J&K)	Coarse and hairy	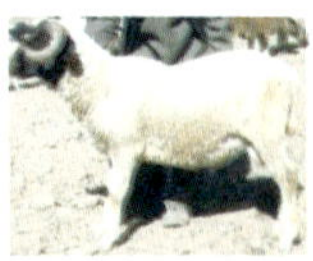
14.	Hassan	Karnataka	Small	Extremely coarse and open	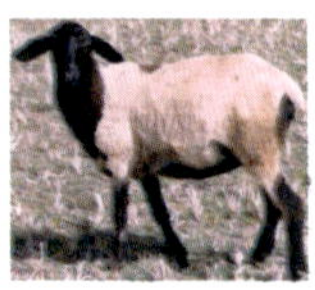

15.	Jaisalmeri	Rajasthan	Large	Medium carpet quality and not very dense	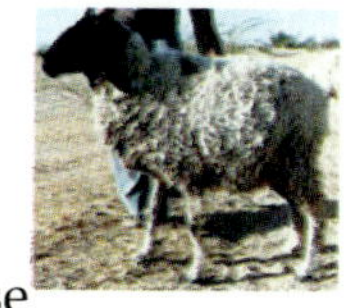
16.	Jalauni	Uttar Pradesh and Madhya Pradesh	Medium	Coarse, short-stapled and open, generally white	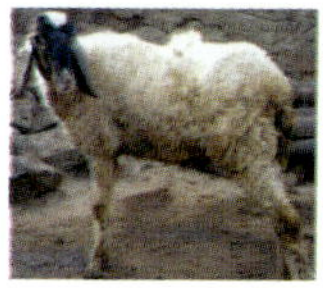
17.	Karnah	Jammu and Kashmir	Large	Coarse and generally white in colour	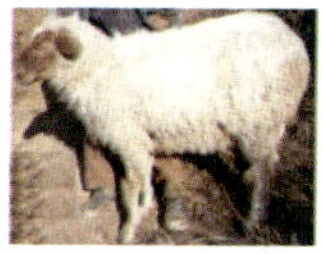
18.	Kenguri (Tenguri)	Karnataka	Medium	Very coarse, hairy meat type breed	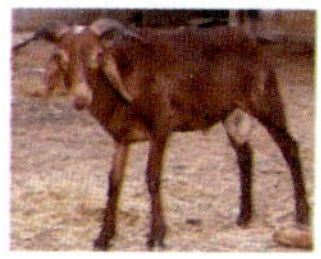
19.	Kilakaraisal (Keezhak-karaisal, Karuvai, Keezha-karauvai, Ramnadkaruvi, Adikaraisal)	Tamil Nadu	Medium	Very coarse, hairy meat type breed	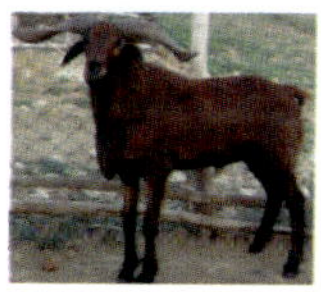
20.	Madras Red	Tamil Nadu	Medium	Body is covered with very short hair which is not shorn	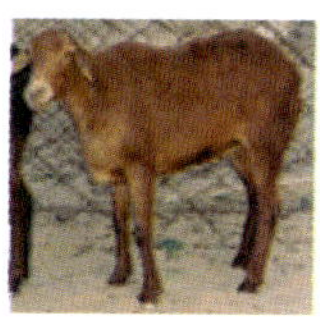
21.	Magra (Bikaneri, Bikaneri Chokla, Chakri)	Rajasthan	Medium	Medium carpet quality, not very dense	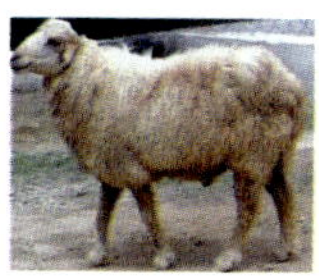

22.	Malpura	Rajasthan	Large	Extremely coarse and hairy	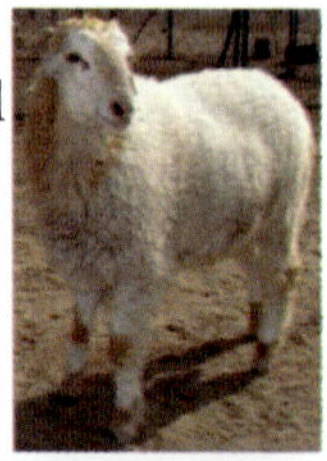
23.	Mandya (Bannur, Bandur)	Karnataka	Small	Extremely coarse and hairy	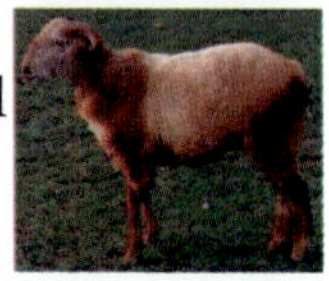
24.	Marwari	Rajasthan and Gujarat	Medium	White and not very dense	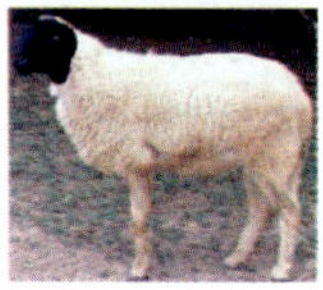
25.	Mecheri (Maiylambadi, Thuvaram-chambali)	Tamil Nadu	Medium	Very short hairs which are not shorn. The is of the highest quality of sheep breeds in India	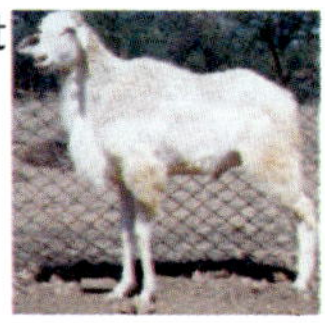
26.	Muzaffar-nagri (Buland-shahri)	Uttar Pradesh and Uttarakhand	Medium to large	White, coarse and open	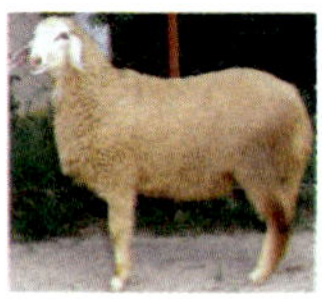
27.	Nali	Rajasthan	Medium	White, coarse, dense and long-stapled	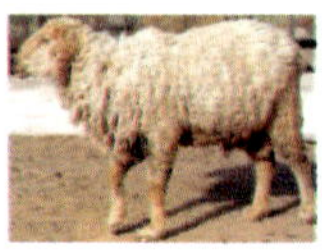
28.	Nellore	Andhra Pradesh	Large	Very coarse, hairy	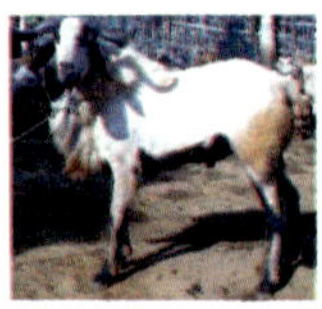

29.	Nilgiri	Tamil Nadu	Medium	Fine and dense	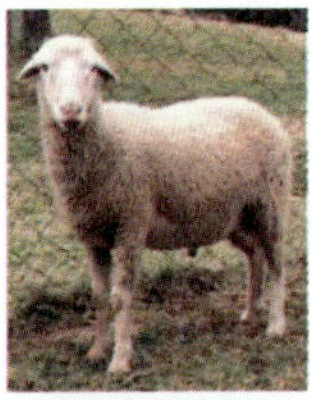
30.	Patanwadi (Desi, Kutchi, Kathiawari, Vadhiyari, Charotari)	Gujarat	Medium to large	Fine to coarse fleece	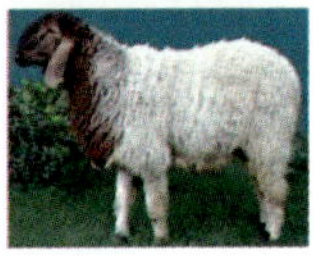
31.	Poonchi	Jammu and Kashmir	Small	Medium to fine quality	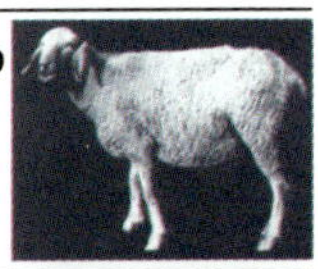
32.	Pugal	Rajasthan	Medium	White and coarse	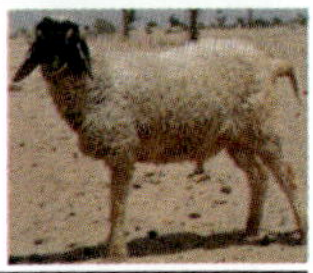
33.	Ramnad White	Tamil Nadu	Medium		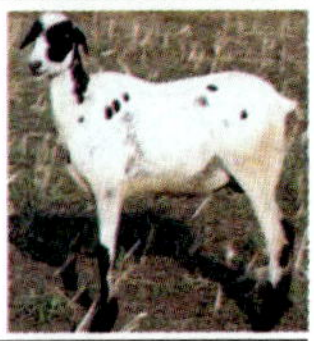
34.	Rampur Bushair	Himachal Pradesh	Medium	Medium quality and dense	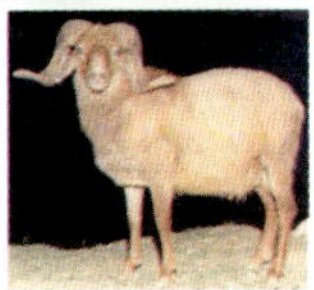
35.	Shahbadi	Bihar	Medium	Extremely coarse, hairy and open	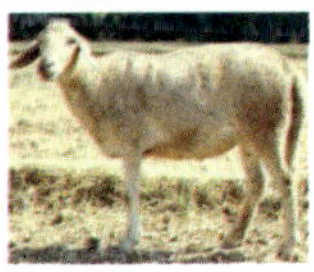
36.	Sonadi	Rajasthan	Large	Extremely coarse and hairy	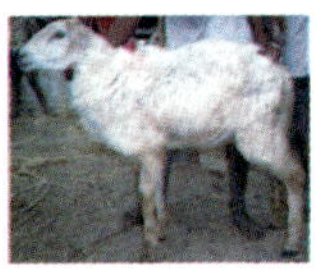
37.	Tibetan	Arunachal Pradesh	Medium	Relatively fine and dense	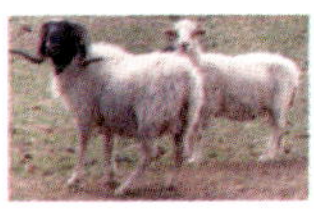

38. Tiruchi Black (Tiruchi Karungurmbai)	Tamil Nadu	Small	Extremely coarse, hairy and open	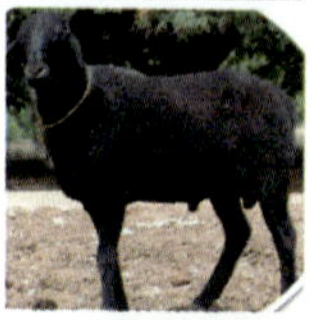
39. Vembur (Karnadhai)	Tamil Nadu		Body is covered with very short hair which is not shorn	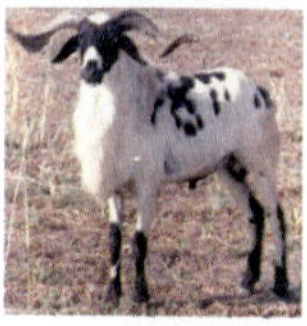
40. Katchaikatty Black	Tamil Nadu	Medium	Coarse and hairy	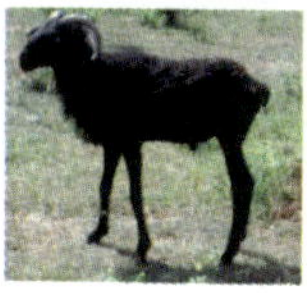

Source: http://www.cswri.res.in/breed_profiles.asp; http://sheepfarm.in/sheep-breeds-gallery; http://agrifarming.in/indian-sheep-breeds; https://sites.google.com/site/viveklpm/sheep-and-goat-production-management/sheep-breeds; http://sapplpp.org/interactive-maps/registered-sheep-breeds-of-india; http://www.nbagr.res.in/Katchaikatty.html; http://www.fao.org/docrep/004/x6532e/X6532E06.htm#ch5.2.4

Some other lesser known goat germplasm need to be explored for production potential

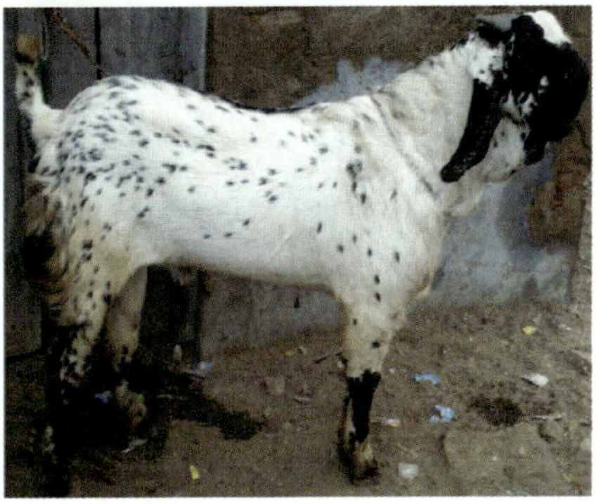

Nagfani buck

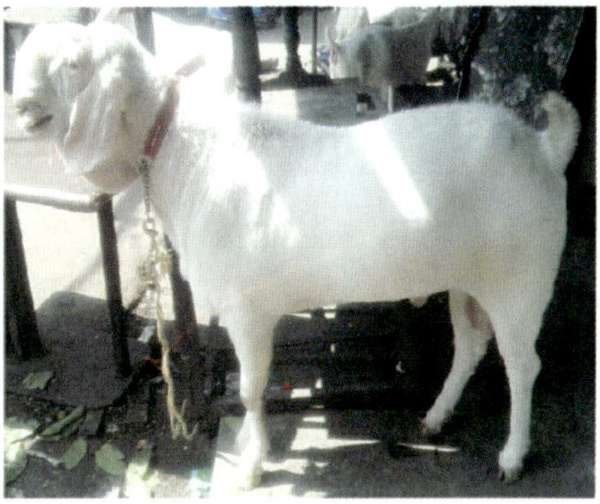

Patira buck

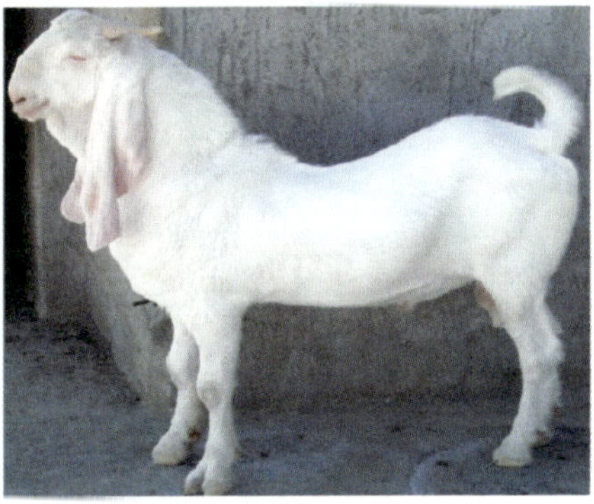

Hyderabadi buck

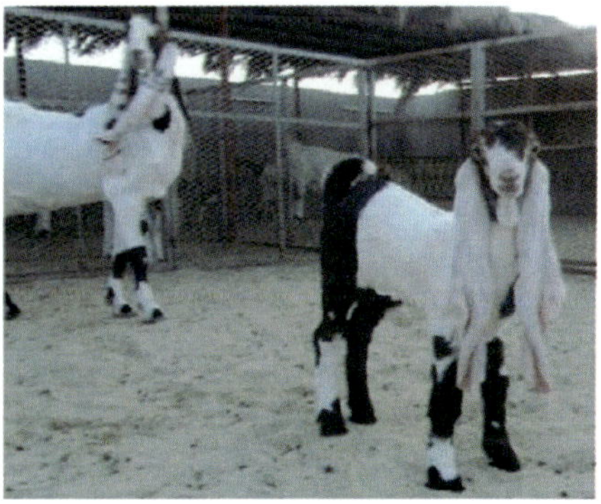

Hyderabadi doe with kid

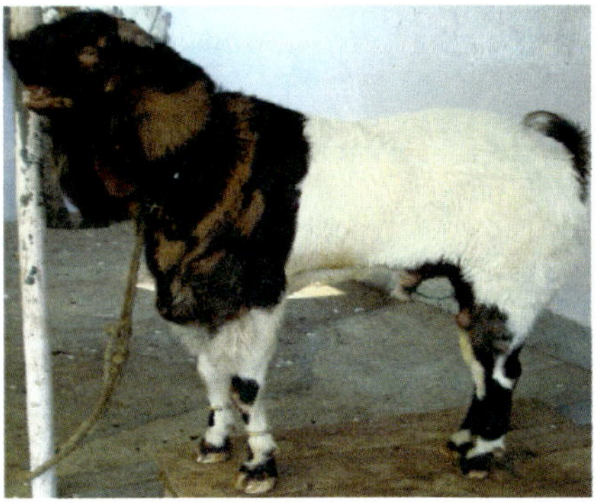

Totapari buck

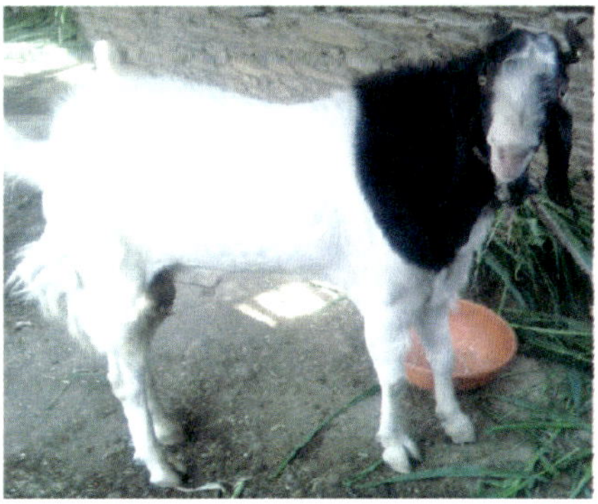

Kota buck

(*Courtsey:* Mr. Naeem Quereshi, Goat supplier, Farah, Mathura)

Table : List of lesser known Sheep germplasm (breeds/strains/varieties) of India

S. No.	Name	Home Tract	Type
1.	Biangi/Kangra Valley	Kangra, Himachal Pradesh	Meat and Wool
2.	Lohi/Parkhanni	Punjab	Wool, Meat and Milk
3.	Bagri	Bagar tract around Delhi	Meat and Carpet wool
4.	Tepli	Pali, Rajasthan	Meat, Milk and Manure
5.	Baradi	Malwa, Madhya Pradesh	-
6.	Danapuri	Uttar Pradesh	-
7.	Marathwada	Maharashtra	Meat
8.	Sangola/Solhapuri	Maharashtra	Meat, Wool, Skin, Manure and Milk
9.	Kolhapuri	Maharashtra	Meat, Wool, Skin, Manure and Milk
10.	Lonand	Maharashtra	Meat, Wool, Skin, Manure and Milk
11.	Sangamneri	Maharashtra	Meat, Wool, Skin, Manure and Milk
12.	Berari	Maharashtra	Meat and Manure
13.	Madgyal	Maharashtra	Meat
14.	Godavari	Maharashtra and Andhra Pradesh	Meat, Milk and Manure
15.	Palla	Andhra Pradesh	Meat
16.	Jodipi/Jodimpu	Andhra Pradesh	Meat
17.	Dora	Andhra Pradesh	Meat
18.	Telingana/Navargade	Andhra Pradesh	Wool
19.	Kattupakkam/ Red sheep	Tamil Nadu	Meat and Skin

20.	MooliKadhu	Tamil Nadu	Meat and Manure
21.	NariKadhu	Tamil Nadu	Meat and Manure
22.	ElaiKadhu	Tamil Nadu	Meat and Manure
23.	Chevaad	Tamil Nadu	-
24.	Dakshini	Odisha	Wool
25.	Kuzi/Desi	Odisha	Meat, Skin and Manure
26.	Edka/Erka	Odisha	Meat, Skin and Manure
27.	Dalua/Red Ganjam	Odisha	Meat, Skin and Manure
28.	Koraput/ Dongriamendha/ Tikriamendha	Odisha	Meat, Skin and Manure
29.	Kendrapada	Odisha	Meat and Skin
30.	Hill sheep	Odisha	Meat, Manure and Skin
31.	Dashamantpur	Odisha	Meat, Manure and Skin
32.	Machhkund	Odisha	Meat, Manure and Skin
33.	Dharamagarh	Odisha	-
34.	Monpa	Arunachal Pradesh	-

(Compiled from Bhatia and Arora, 2010)

□□□

Chapter 6

CONCLUDING REMARKS

Proper utilization of sheep and goat genetic resources is most important and need much emphasis to be put on the productivity characteristics, while the surveys are being made for collection of information of breeds. There is a wide gap between production potential and present productivity in small ruminants of the county and existing genetic diversity provide great scope for their development. Small ruminants with better performance above the flock average should be identified and utilized for improvement programmes by organizing open nucleus breeding schemes. It is necessary to improve the prevailing management efforts and technologies for appropriate management of sheep and goat genetic resources in India. There is the need to develop, improve and make sustainable use of genetic resources using multidisciplinary approach with a farming system perceptive.

Considering the production potential of small ruminants in view of climatic changes, specially goat rearing is shifting from a livelihood activity for poor and landless farmers to a full-fledged commercial enterprise. While establishing the sheep and goat farm in commercial way, the farmers have been purchasing recognized breeds at higher price per kilogram live weight on the basis of breed name from their home tract and transporting them for long distance which poses high mortality due to transport stress and poor management. It has been observed at CIRG over the time after analyzing the reasons for gradual closure of commercial farms immediately after the establishment and found that the poor foundation stock and preference of known breeds from distant places are the main reasons for such closures. Moreover, brokers/middlemen are cheating the small ruminant keepers by claiming the less known/nondescript breed as recognized breed of

India and fetch more prices in the name of breed. Hence the knowledge on the performance of these lesser known small ruminant germplasm will help the sheep and goat keepers to buy the known/less known sheep and goats available nearer to them to avoid such initial major losses and it may not demotivate the farmers who want to establish the sheep and goats farming in commercial way in future.

❑❑❑

REFERENCES

19th Livestock Census. 2012. All India Report. Ministry of Agriculture, Department of Animal Husbandry, Dairying and Fisheries, Krishi Bhawan, New Delhi.

Annual Report. 2008-09. Assam Hill goat. ICAR Research Complex for NEH Region, Umiam-793 103, Meghalaya

Annual Report. 2009-10. Assam Hill goat. ICAR Research Complex for NEH Region, Umiam-793 103, Meghalaya

Annual Report. 2010-11. Assam Hill goat. ICAR Research Complex for NEH Region, Umiam-793 103, Meghalaya.

Annual Report, NBAGR 2010-11. Bundelkhandi and Berari goats. National Bureau of Animal Genetic Resources, Karnal. pp 14-16.

Anthra 2006. Livestock based livelihood- an action programme for the Andaman and Nicobar Islands. Proceedings of seminar, 13-24 November 2006, Port Blair, Andamans.

Barwal, R. S., Singh, C. V. and Singh, S. 2010a. Udaipuri Goat-A newly found animal genetic resource in the western Himalayan region of Uttarakhand. Abstract No. B31. National Symposium on challenges to domestic Animal Biodiversity and Action Plan for its Management and Utilization. 10-11 Feb., Anand Agricultural University, Anand. pp 127-28.

Barwal, R. S., Singh, C. V. and Singh, S. 2010b. Characterization of Udaipuri goat in semi temperate region of western Uttarakhand. Abstract No. B4. National Symposium on challenges to domestic Animal Biodiversity & Action Plan for its Management and Utilization. 10-11 Feb., Anand Agricultural University, Anand. pp 113.

Basic Animal Husbandry and Fisheries Statistics 2014; Government of India Ministry of Agriculture Department of Animal Husbandry, Dairying and Fisheries Krishi Bhawan, New Delhi.

Bhatia, S. and Arora, R. 2010.Lesser known ovine germplasm-An under evaluated asset of India. *Indian Journal of Animal Sciences* 80(9): 880-890.

Bhusan, S., Charanjeet Kaur and Hemant Kumar. 2010. Goats in Bundelkhand region. Abstract No. B12. National Symposium on challenges to domestic Animal Biodiversity and Action Plan for its Management and Utilization. 10-11 Feb., Anand Agricultural University, Anand. pp 117-118.

Bhusan, S., Charanjeet Kaur, Vijay Bahadur and Hemant Kumar. 2010. Performance of Bundelkhand and goats in draught conditions. Abstract No. B30. National Symposium on challenges to domestic Animal Biodiversity and Action Plan for its Management and Utilization. 10-11 Feb., Anand Agricultural University, Anand. pp 127.

Das, N. 2008. Bareilly goat - A potential strain for meat production. Proceeding of National Symposium on Redefining role of indigenous animal genetic resources in rural development held on 15-16 February, 2008 at Karnataka Veterinary, Animal and Fisheries Science University, Bidar.

Devendra, C. and Burns, M. 2000. Goat Production in the Tropics. Commonwealth Agricultural Bureaux, United Kingdom, pp. 49-54.

Ekambaram, B., Gupta, B. R., Prakash, M. G. and Sudhaker, K. 2011c. Reproductive performance of Mahabubnagar goats under field conditions. *Indian Veterinary Journal* 88(12): 38-40.

Ekambaram, B., Gupta, B. R., Prakash, M. G., Sudhaker, K and Reddy, V. R. 2011a. Morphological characterization of Mahabubnagar goats. *Indian Journal of Animal Sciences* 81 (2): 176–179.

Ekambaram, B., Gupta, B. R., Prakash, M. G., Sudhaker, K and Reddy, V. R. 2011b. Housing, breeding and management practices of Mahabubnagar goats. *Indian Journal of Animal Sciences* 81 (8): 176–179.

Ekambaram, B., Ramesh B. Gupta, Prakash M. Gnana, Sudhaker, K. and Reddy, V. R. 2010. A study on the performance of Mahabubnagar goats. *Indian Journal of Animal Research* 44 (1): 48-51.

F.A.O. Statistics. 1999. The global strategy for the management of farm animal genetic resources. Executive Brief Rome part 4: State of the art in the management of animal genetic resources. ftp://ftp. fao. org / crep/fao/ meeting/012/ah834e /ah834e04.pdf.

F.A.O. Statistics. 2010. www.fao.org/FAOSTAT. Food and Agricultural Organisation of the United Nations. Rome.

F.A.O. Statistics. 2013. www.fao.org /FAOSTAT. Food and Agricultural Organisation of the United Nations. Rome.

Jain, A., Sahana, G., Kandasamy, N. and Nivsarkar, A.E. 2000. Kodi Adu- A new goat breed of Tamil Nadu. *Indian Journal of Animal Sciences* 70 (6): 649-651.

Jeyakumar, S, Jai Sunder, Yadav, S.P. and Kundu, A. 2000. Characterization conservation evaluation and improvement of native Teressa Goat- An unreported indigenous germ plasm (http://cari.res.in/animal-ach/teressa%20 goat.htm).

Jindal S. K. 1984. Goat Production. Falcon Books from Cosmo publication, New Delhi, India.

Joshi, B.P. 1992. A new goat strain in semi temperate central Himalayan region. In: Pre conference proceedings, Abstracts of contributory papers, Volume I: V International conference on goats. New Delhi p20.

Kornel, D., Mohapatra, S.C. and Acharya, R.M. 2006. Sheep and goat genetic resources of Orissa. A survey Report with Government of Orissa through Indo Swiss Natural Resource Management Programme. Inter cooperation India delegation, Hyderabad. pp 1-118.

Kundu M.S., De A.K., Jeyakumar S., Sunder J., Kundu A. and Sujatha T. 2014. Effect of zinc supplementation on reproductive performance of Teressa goat. *Veterinary World*, 7 (6):380-383.

Kundu, A., Sunder, J., Jeyakumar, S., Verma, S.K., Kundu, M.S., De, A.K. and Srivastava, R.C. 2010. Livestock and poultry production policy for Andaman and Nicobar Islands: A scientific perspective. Published by Director, CARI, Port Blair. p1-48.

Mane, S. H., Mandakmale, S. D., Kankhare, D. H. and Dhage S. A. 2015. Kathewadi goat: A boon to hilly areas of Khandesh region of Maharastra. Abstract No. TS-I-31. International Symposium on Sustainable management of animal genetic resources for livelihood security in developing countries & XII Annual Convention of SOCDAB. February 13-14, Madras Veterinary College, Chennai. pp 68-69.

Manson, I. L. 1998. A World Dictionary of Livestock Breeds. 3rd Edn., C.A.B. International Publication, Wallingfor Oxon (UK), pp. 125.

Mariadas, B. 1996. Tamil Nattin Velladu Inangal (Goats Breeds of Tamil Nadu) pp.1-13.

Mishra, P., Ali, A. S. and Verma, N. K. 2012 Phenotypic, biometric and genetic characterization of Bundelkhandi goats. *Indian Journal of Animal Sciences* 82 (11): 1442–45.

Mohanty, G. P., Das, S. and Mohapatra, S. P. 2011. Production performance of Kalahandi goats in its native tract. Abstract No. T2.18. Proceedings of National Symposium on Animal genetic resources for Sustainable Livestock Sector in India, 18-19th February at Bhubaneswar, Odisha. pp 137-138.

Patro, B. N., Nayak, S., Rao, P. K. and Panda, P. 2007. Genetic studies of Ghumusar goats of Orissa. *Indian Journal of Animal Breeding and Genetics* 27: 12-16.

Raja, K. N., Navneet Kaur, Anand Jain and Joshi, B. K. 2011. Adilabad Black, an unexplored goat germplasm. Abstract No. SS1-13. In: Compendium of lead papers and abstracts of National seminar on Sheep and Goat Production held at Sheep Breeding Research Station of TANUVAS, Sandynallah, The Nilgiris from 28-29th December 2011. pp 26.

Ravimurugan, T., Devendran, P., Cauveri, D. and Balachandran, S. 2009. Performance of indigenous goat (*Pallai Adu*) under field conditions. *Tamil Nadu Journal of Veterinary and Animal Sciences* 5 (5): 203-207.

Roy, B. G., Roy, U., Gogei, D. and Ahmed. 2007. Non-pashmina goat of Ladakh: A note. In: Proceeding of National Symposium on 'Role of animal genetic resources in rural livelihood security'. 8-9 February, 2007 at Birsa Agricultural University, Ranchi (Jharkhand).

Sadana, D. K. and Kaur, N. 2011. Alternate livestock breed systems for tropical islands in the face of climate change. In: International Conference on Tropical Island Ecosystems: issues related to Livelihood, Sustainable Development and Climate Change held at CARI, Port Blair from 23-26th March 2011. TIECON.

Shettar, V.B. and Rudresh, B.H. 2003a. External features of indigenous Bidri goats. *Indian Veterinary Journal* 80: 941-942.

Shettar, V. B. and Rudresh, B. H. 2003b. Body measurements of Bidri goats. *Indian Veterinary Journal* 80: 367-368.

Singh, C. V. and Barwal, R. S. 2007. Chaugarkha goat - a unique strain of goat in central Himalayan ecosystem. *Indian Journal of Small Ruminants* 13(1): 61-64.

Singh, C. V. and Barwal, R. S. 2009. Characterization of Chaugarkha goats in their home tract. *Indian Journal of Small Ruminants* 15(2): 274-76.

Singh, C. V., Barwal, R. S. and Singh, C. B. 2010. Domestic animal biodiversity and breeding policy for genetic up gradation of livestock of Uttarakhand. Lead Paper in National symposium on challenges to Domestic Animal Biodiversity and Action Plan for its Management and Utilization. 10-11 Feb. 2010, Anand Agricultural University, Anand. pp 48-53.

Singh, M. K., Dixit A. K., Roy A. K. and Singh S. K. 2014. Analysis of prospects and problems of goat production in Bundelkhand region. *Range Management and Agroforestry* 35 (1): 163-168

Singh, M. K., Dige M. S. and Dixit A. K. 2014. Dudharu bakri ki nayi nasal: Battisi. *Goat News*. 29 : 11.

Singh, V. K., Singh, N. S., Kumar, P. and Patel, A. K. 2010a. Phenotypic characterization of Jaunpuri goats in its native tracts. Abstract No. B8. National Symposium on challenges to domestic Animal biodiversity and action plan for its management and utilization. 10-11 Feb., 2010, Anand Agricultural university, Anand. pp 115.

Singh, V. K., Singh, N. S., Patel, A. K. and Kumar, P. 2010b. Evaluation of some economic traits of Jaunpuri goats of eastern Uttar Pradesh. Abstract No. B19. National Symposium on challenges to domestic Animal Biodiversity & Action Plan for its Management and Utilization. 10-11 Feb., 2010, Anand Agricultural university, Anand. pp 121.

Srivastava S.P. and Saraswat B.L. 2006. Marketing of Jaunpuri goats in its native tract. *Indian Journal of Animal Research.* 40 (2): 127-130.

Thilagam, K., Ramamoorthy, J., Sivaselvam, S. N., Karthickeyan, S. M. K. and Thangaraju, P. 2011. Molecular genetic characterization of Salem Black goats *(Capra hircus)* using microsatellite markers. Abstract No. SS3-18. In: Compendium of lead papers and abstracts of National seminar on sheep and goat production held at Sheep Breeding Research Station of TANUVAS, Sandynallah, The Nilgiris from 28-29th December 2011. pp 114.

Thiruvenkadan, A. K. 2012. Kodi Adu-A Monograph. International Foundation for Science and Tamilnadu Veterinary and Animal Sciences University, Chennai, Tamil Nadu. P 1-87.

Thiruvenkadan, A. K. and Karunanithi, K. 2006. Characterization of Salem Black goats in their home tract. *Animal Genetic Resources Information* 38: 67-75.

Verma, N. K., Dixit, S. P., Dangi, P. S., Aggarwal, R. A. K., Das, S. K., Mishra P. and Tyagi, N. 2011. Phenotypic characterization of Ghumsari goat of Odisha. Abstract No. T2.21. Proceedings of National Symposium on Animal genetic resources for sustainable livestock sector in india, 18-19th February at Bhubaneswar, Odisha. pp 139-40.

Verma, N. K., Dangi, P. S., Dixit, S. P., Aggarwal, R. A. K., Das, S. K. 2013. Morphologic and biometric study of Malkangiri goats of Odisha. Proceedings of National Symposium on Integrated development of vast biodiversity of indigenous livestock for long term rural livelihood security, 7-8th February at GBPAU&T, Uttrakhand. pp 262-63.

Verma, N. K., Kaur, N. and Mishra, P. 2010. Lesser known goat population-Need for their characterization and recognition. *Journal of Livestock Biodiversity* 2 (1): 1-6.

Verma, N. K., Mishra, P., Aggarwal, R. A. K., Dixit, S. P., Dangi, P. S. And Das, S. K. 2015. Characterisation, performance and genetic diversity among goats of odisha. *Indian Journal of Animal Sciences* 85 (2): 165-171.

Verma, N. K., Aggarwal, R. A. K., Sharma, R., Dangi, P. S. and Bhutia, N. T. 2015. Phenotypic characterisation, biometry and management of Singharey goat of Sikkim. *Indian Journal of Animal Sciences* 85 (7): 810-812.

Yadav, S. P. Jeyakumar, S., Jai Sunder, and Kundu, A. 2000. Conservation and phenotypic and molecular characterization of indigenous goats of Andaman and Nicobar islands. http://cari.res.in/animal-ach/conservation%20and%20 phenotypic %20 goats.htm

Zeshmarani, S., Dhara, K. C., Samanta, A. K., Samanta, R. and Majumder, S. C. 2007. Reproductive performance of goats in Eastern and North-eastern India. *Livestock Research and Rural Development*, 19: Article 114.

http://sojatgoatsindia.blogspot.ae/2011/03/sojat-goats-in-india.html).

http://www.vivekamfarms.com/goat_farming/goat_breeds/karoli;

http://www.al-nwader.com/vb/t6342.html).

❑❑❑